Handbook of Vacuum
Extraction in Obstetric Practice

DEDICATION

To all mothers and their babies,
especially Janet and hers

Handbook of Vacuum Extraction in Obstetric Practice

Aldo Vacca MB BS, FRANZCOG, FRCOG, GCEd

Clinical Associate Professor
Department of Obstetrics and Gynaecology
The University of Queensland

Director of Obstetric Services
Caboolture Hospital
Queensland, Australia

Vacca Research
BRISBANE

© 1997 Aldo Vacca

First published in Great Britain 1992
Reprinted in Australia 1999

British Library Cataloguing in Publication Data
Vacca, Aldo
 Handbook of Vacuum Extraction in
 Obstetric Practice
 I. Title
 618.8

 ISBN 0–340–54849–5

Whilst the advice and information in this book is believed to be true
and accurate at the date of going to press, neither the author nor the
publisher can accept any legal responsibility or liability for any errors
or omissions that may be made. In particular (but without limiting the
generality of the preceding disclaimer) every effort has been made to
check drug dosages; however, it is still possible that errors have been
missed. Furthermore, dosage schedules are constantly being revised
and new side effects recognised. For these reasons the reader is
strongly urged to consult the drug companies' printed instructions
before administering any of the drugs recommended in this book.

CONTENTS

FOREWORD

The vacuum extractor holds an interesting place in world opinion. In some countries it has replaced the obstetric forceps, in others it is hardly ever used. Both these opinions owe more to the heart than the head for the vacuum extractor is a most valuable instrument and should never be considered an alternative to forceps. The two have different indications and different usages; perhaps more important, the two have entirely different sets of skills, both of which should be learned and practised by a working obstetrician for either method may be needed in an emergency.

This volume gives an up to date account of the vacuum extractor from a country where its use is common. Dr Vacca is an experienced obstetrician with the double skill of also being a good teacher. In consequence, this volume clearly and logically follows through the material that anyone who wanted to know about vacuum extraction could read. It can be used at two levels: by the doctors and midwives who wish to perform vacuum ex-traction and also with great effect by those who are training for higher degrees and wish to be able to answer questions of the examiners on the theory and practice of the ventouse. Throughout, the author emphasizes that it is not the instrument that will compensate for any clinical deficiencies; it is only the tool in the hands of the person who must assess the situation correctly before applying either vacuum or forceps.

This book is thoroughly recommended to all with an interest in practical obstetrics: they will have to use the vacuum extractor, therefore they may as well use it with full knowledge which Dr Vacca would provide.

Geoffrey Chamberlain RD MD FRCS FRCOG
FACOG(Hon)
Professor of Obstetrics
University of London
at St George's Hospital Medical School

PREFACE

Controversy still surrounds the use of the obstetric vacuum extractor as a means of assisting a woman to give birth. So many differing opinions have been expressed about the value and safety of this instrument that it is not surprising some users and would-be users are uncertain of its place in current obstetric practice. Conflicting opinions are held as to whether the vacuum extractor should be used before the cervix is fully dilated; whether the method is safe at higher stations of the head than is generally accepted for forceps; and whether the instrument is effective for the management of malpositions of the fetal head. There is disagreement, too, about whether the vacuum should be induced rapidly or slowly; whether the duration of the procedure precludes its use when the fetus is distressed, and whether detachment of the cup should be regarded as a safety feature or a cause of scalp injury. This handbook sets out, by addressing these controversies, to help clinicians develop a balanced view about the value of this instrument in modern obstetrics.

The book is also designed to assist clinicians sift through the confusion that may be caused by the proliferation of vacuum cups manufactured in a variety of designs, materials and sizes. Unless operators understand the reasons why these modifications have been introduced and know how to adjust their technique according to the type of cup that is used, the potential benefits of the design will not be fully realized.

There are strongly held views about the relative merits and limitations of vacuum extraction compared to forceps delivery. Regional and international variations in the choice of instrument for operative vaginal delivery have more to do with tradition than choice based on evaluation of the relative merits. In theory, the two instruments may be regarded as interchangeable for most of the indications for operative vaginal delivery but, because operative technique is different for the two instruments, experience gained in one method does not automatically transfer to the other. Although this book focuses on the benefits of the vacuum extractor when properly used, some claims about the relative value and safety of the instrument must be interpreted with caution. The reader's attention is drawn to some of the problems surrounding the evidence on which these claims are based.

It should be appreciated that, as with forceps delivery, the instrument is only one of a number of factors that contribute to the overall success or failure of vacuum extraction. Dilatation of the cervix, station and position of the head, and the condition of the fetus and mother will, either singly or in combination influence the outcome to a varying degree. The book shows how these factors must be carefully evaluated in every case to decide which method of operative delivery is most appropriate in the circumstances. When the instrument of choice is the vacuum extractor, the next important variable to consider is technique. Correct technique is essential for good results with the vacuum extractor; incorrect technique is unlikely to injure the mother but may seriously injure the baby. Many studies have reported a range of complications associated with vacuum extraction, but few have attempted to identify the predisposing factors or underlying causes. This book, by stressing correct technique and by developing preventive measures and guidelines, should enable operators to avoid the pitfalls frequently associated with the vacuum extractor.

These are some of the issues that the handbook

addresses. Although it has been written primarily for obstetricians (and midwives) who use or intend to use the vacuum extractor and for those who are responsible for teaching the technique, the book is also directed at a much wider group of health professionals. Obstetricians in training and obstetricians who have traditionally preferred the forceps but who are considering using the vacuum extractor should find the information in this handbook helpful to understand the essential principles of vacuum extraction and how proper technique differs between the two instruments. Neonatal paediatricians and nurses, and midwives who attend mothers during labour and after birth should also find the information in the handbook of value, as should all care-givers who are privileged to assist women in childbirth.

A Vacca
Brisbane, 1991

ACKNOWLEDGEMENTS

In one way or another, colleagues and friends in various parts of the world have encouraged the author to produce this book. It would not have been completed, however, without the dedicated effort of a select group of people. Special thanks is due to Kerri Nelson, medical artist, whose skill and ability to grasp the principles, transformed the author's ideas and sketches into the clear illustrations presented in the book. I am indebted to Vicki Adams and to members of the Mater Misericordiae Hospitals' Photography Department for their assistance in the preparation of the illustrations for reproduction, and to Avon Simpson and Sharon Taylor who patiently typed and retyped the numerous drafts of the manuscript. Finally, I would like to express my thanks to the editorial staff of Edward Arnold for their support and advice throughout the project.

1

EQUIPMENT

DEVELOPMENT OF THE MODERN OBSTETRIC VACUUM EXTRACTORS

The obstetric vacuum extractor, sometimes called the ventouse is an instrument which, like the forceps, may be used to assist a woman to give birth. Essentially all vacuum extractors consist of a cup made of rigid or soft material, a traction device and a vacuum system that provides negative pressure suction by which the cup is attached to the fetal scalp. Vacuum extraction as an effective alternative to the obstetric forceps as a method to assist a woman to give birth was introduced less than half a century ago, although the concept for the technique is much older. Excellent reviews of the history of vacuum extraction may be found in the monographs of Dragotescu[1] and Chalmers[2].

Rigid (metal) cups

Malmstrom cups

Malmstrom[3] of Gothenburg is generally acknowledged as the 'father' of the modern vacuum extractor. In 1952, he took up the challenge of devising an effective obstetric vacuum extractor and, in 1957, introduced the system which is still used today in a form little changed from the original design. The main feature of this instrument has been the unique design of the vacuum cup which has formed the basis for all other metal cup modifications. The Malmstrom vacuum extractor (Fig. 1.1) has the cup in the shape of a flattened hollow hemisphere whose margins are incurved so that the diameter across the opening is smaller than the greatest diameter of the cup. As a result, when the cup is applied to the fetal scalp

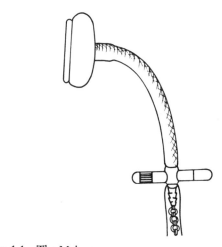

Fig. 1.1 The Malmstrom cup

and a suitable vacuum is induced, an artificial caput succedaneum called the chignon is formed. When this fills the cup, the edge of the opening of the cup underlies the greatest diameter of the caput so that a substantial traction force may be applied without causing detachment. The margin of the cup has been rounded in order to reduce the risk of injury to the scalp.

Malmstrom's cup is characterized by having the suction tubing attached to a short metal pipe on the centre of the dome of the cup and the traction chain passing through the middle of the tubing.

The following advantages were claimed for the Malmstrom cup:

- considerable traction force could be generated
- there was no need to pass the instrument around the fetal head

– traction could be either synchronous with uterine contractions and maternal expulsive effort to enable delivery to be completed in a shorter time or could be continuous with a weak traction
– the instrument could be used to alter the position of the fetal head and so modify the presenting diameters
– the direction of the traction could be varied
– the instrument could be used with the fetal head at high or low stations in the pelvis
– the instrument could be used for maternal and fetal indications
– the instrument was safe for both mother and baby.

Users of the Malmstrom device soon recognized that there was a tendency for the cup to become dislodged when the direction of traction was oblique [4, 5, 6, 7, 8]. When traction was applied at an acute angle to Malmstrom's cup, the metal pipe for the suction tube on the dome of the cup (Fig. 1.2a) behaved as a lever and the cup tended to tilt and detach from the fetal scalp (Fig. 1.2b). Such leverage does not readily occur if traction is applied at right angles to the cup but this direction is not always ideal obstetrically. It also became apparent that manoeuvrability of the Malmstrom cup within the introitus was restricted by the suction tube meeting the vulval tissues at the entrance of the vagina and that it was sometimes impossible to position the cup correctly over the ideal site especially in malpositions of the fetal head[9]. For these reasons, various modifications to the original Malmstrom design were made, in order to increase the cup's manoeuvrability or to reduce the tendency for detachment.

Variations on the Malmstrom cup

Sjostedt[10] altered the Malmstrom cup by shortening the metal suction pipe by 4 mm and setting it into a depression on the surface of the cup so that it projected only 4 mm above the dome. While this made application easier, obliquely applied traction still tended to lever the cup off the fetal scalp. Modifications were also made to the traction system with the introduction of a T-shaped traction handle which could be attached to the tube by threading it through a series of hooks and notches. However the fitting of the traction handle could be difficult and time consuming, and the application

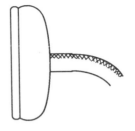

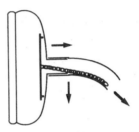

Fig. 1.2(a) and (b)   The leverage factor. With oblique traction the point of action is transferred to the end of the suction pipe
(Fig. 1.2(b) has been reproduced from Bird: 'Modification of Malmstrom's vacuum extractor'. *British Medical Journal*. 1969; **3**, 525, by kind permission of the author and publishers)

of traction frequently led to detachment of the tubing. Consequently, this mechanism has not become popular. Halkin[6] addressed the tilt factor by displacing the vacuum tube attachment from the centre of the cup to the periphery of the dome and also by depressing the middle of the surface to achieve a reduction in the cup's central height from 50 to 10 mm. Laboratory testing of the Halkin model proved the theoretic consideration to be correct; at a traction angle of 30 degrees the loss of effective traction force amounted to 6 per cent compared to 47 per cent when the Malmstrom device was used. Halkin's cup has not been developed for clinical use.

Lovset[7] designed a cup with a new type of traction apparatus which he described as follows:

'To prevent the cup from turning over by side traction, 4 holes were made for fastening nooses on 2 loops of cord. To each of these loops, a block was attached and from each of the blocks went a third loop with a third block. This arrangement distributed traction evenly around the periphery of the suction cup and minimized the tendency to slip off when side traction was applied.'

Lovset also flattened the edge of the cup on one side and moved the suction tube from the centre to the periphery of the dome, giving this tube an oblique attachment to the surface. With a negative pressure of 0.51 kg/cm² and a traction angle of 45 degrees, Lovset claimed that his cup withstood a pull of 9 kgms while Malmstrom's cup of the same size withstood a pull of 3.7 kgms. Lovset's cup has not been introduced into clinical practice.

Party[11] introduced a commercial suction cup made of rigid plastic material that he called the ventouse obstetricale française. The cup had the general design of the Malmstrom cup but the suction attachment was eccentric. The traction system consisted of a flexible handle connected to the centre of the cup by a universal joint. Saling[12] developed a modification of the traction system by attaching a handle to the top of the cup through a joint that allowed the handle to be laid horizontal to the dome. He claimed that this modification facilitated insertion and application of the cup and allowed the direction of traction to be oblique. However, it did not eliminate the tendency for cup detachment with oblique pulls. Drapier[13] developed a 'minicup' that was claimed to have advantages because of a reduced depth of the cup resulting from the suction system being attached to the lateral wall which allowed the cup to slide more easily over the fetal head and achieve a more correct application. Traction was applied through a flexible wire attached to a bar fixed into a recess in the centre of the dome and attached to a handle set at a variable distance from the cup. Although these cups have been produced commercially, they have not become widely known.

Bird cups

Bird[4] addressed the problem of cup detachment by separating the suction and traction systems, attaching the metal pipe for the suction tube eccentrically on the dome of the cup (Fig. 1.3). Because traction now acted at the level of the surface of the cup and not at the end of the suction nozzle, the length of the 'lever' was effectively reduced to the cup's depth, thus, in theory lessening the tendency to detach from the scalp. This

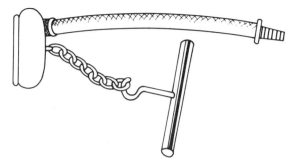

Fig. 1.3 The Bird Anterior cup (original model)

design was originally called the Modified Cup but is now called the anterior cup. With a negative pressure of 0.7 kg/cm² and a traction angle of 45 degrees, this type of cup tested on an artificial scalp withstood a pull of 8.8 kgms. Under identical conditions, Malmstrom's cup withstood 3.8 kgms and Sjostedt's cup 5.8 kgms. With perpendicular traction each cup, 5 cms in diameter, withstood a pull of 11.3 kgms. Bird claimed that his cup had other advantages: preparation for use was very easy and rapidly completed; the eccentric, oblique suction tube did not obstruct the process of application as much as the central vertical tube allowing a better (more posterior) application with this cup than with Malmstrom's cup; the traction apparatus was simpler than Malmstrom's and consisted of a chain and a traction bar with a hook which could pick up a link of the chain at any convenient point.

Bird also recognized that the range of movement of the cup within the introitus depended on the depth of the cup and the attachment of the tubing. Cups with central dome-attached tubing were more restricted in their lateral movement but in many cases even the eccentric suction tube of the modified cup still hindered application to the ideal site on the fetal head when the occiput was posterior[9]. To increase manoeuvrability of the cup, Bird moved the attachment of the suction pipe to the lateral wall so that the tubing, being in the same plane as the body of the cup, should theoretically be less likely to restrict the cup's movements (Fig. 1.4) and allow a more frequent correct application. This design, originally called the OP cup is now known as the Posterior cup and is recommended for use in posterior and lateral positions of the occiput. Bird subsequently modified the traction system of his original Anterior and Posterior cup

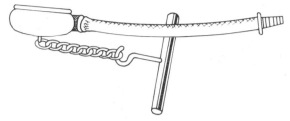

Fig. 1.4   The Bird Posterior cup (original model)

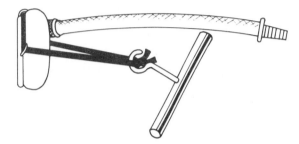

Fig. 1.5   The Bird Anterior cup (New Generation model)

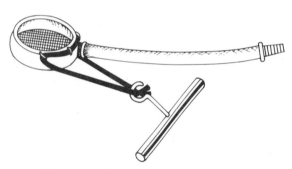

Fig. 1.6   The Bird Posterior cup (New Generation model)

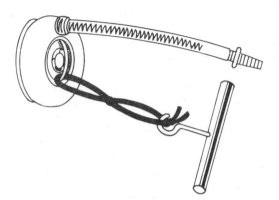

Fig. 1.7   The O'Neil Anterior cup

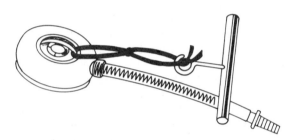

Fig. 1.8   The O'Neil Posterior cup

designs by replacing the chain attached to the dome of the cup with a looped nylon cord attached to the rim. These cord or string cups have been called New Generation Cups and are available in the Anterior (Fig. 1.5) and Posterior (Fig. 1.6) models.

O'Neil cups

O'Neil[8] devised a new traction system which he incorporated into cups with the anterior (Fig. 1.7) and posterior (Fig. 1.8) design patterns. His cups had a circular plate on the dome which rotated on a bearing and to which was attached a metal rod curved to form part of the perimeter of a circle the centre of which was a point in the middle of the opening of the cup (Fig. 1.9). Traction was mediated by a loop of nylon cord around the curved metal rod which allowed the cord to slide along the rod when the direction of pull was oblique. O'Neil claimed that the device had an advantage over other cups in not lifting at one edge even when the direction of traction was oblique because the traction system effectively directed the point of action of pull to the middle of the opening of the cup.

Soft (plastic or silicone) cups

The Soft cups are so named because they are manufactured from pliable silicone or plastic materials. The basic design is bell or trumpet-shaped with a stem attached to the top of the dome which serves as a traction handle and through which the vacuum pipe passes. The cups are modifications of a device introduced by Kobayashi and is similar to the instrument devised by J Y Simp-

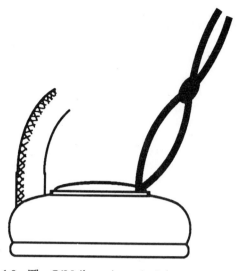

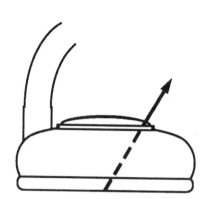

Fig. 1.9 The O'Neil traction principle
(Published with permission of the editor of the *Australian and New Zealand Journal of Obstetrics and Gynaecology*)

son more than a century before[2]. In theory, the rigid central handle and increased depth of the cups would appear to render them less manoeuvrable than the posterior cup models but they may be associated with fewer adverse effects on the baby's scalp[14]. There are four types of soft cups in common use: the Silastic, Silc, Mityvac and CMI cups.

The Silastic cup

The Silastic obstetrical vacuum cup is a trumpet-shaped device made from pliable translucent silicone elastomer (Fig. 1.10). It is claimed that the design of the device and the soft material from which it is constructed enhance its safety and allows it to be easily folded and inserted through the vaginal introitus with minimal risk of injury to the mother; distributes the traction force evenly over the entire occiput thereby reducing the risk of cephalhaematoma and scalp injury; and provides effective attachment even in the presence of a caput succedaneum.

The Silc cup

The Silc cup, introduced in 1984, is made from silicone rubber also in the Kobayashi trumpet-shaped design (Fig. 1.11). The advantages claimed are similar to those of the other soft cups, namely ease of application, effective adherence to the scalp and minimal risk of injury to mother and baby. A low cost version, the Santoprene cup, is sold in some countries and more recently a new design, the short Silc cup, has become available (Fig. 1.12). In this latter cup, the traction system comprises a

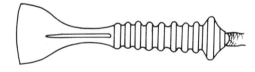

Fig. 1.11 The Silc cup

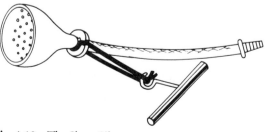

Fig. 1.12 The Short Silc cup

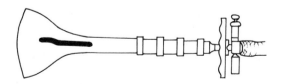

Fig. 1.10 The Silastic cup

looped cord attached to a collar near the top of the cup with a handle hooked into the other end of the loop.

Mityvac cup

The Mityvac obstetrical vacuum cup was the first commercially available plastic cup. It is made in the shape of a bell and is supplied with a light-weight hand pump which, with the cup, forms a unit known as the Obstetrical Vacuum Delivery System. The M-cup, a plastic cup based on the Malmstrom design, is also produced by the same manufacturer.

CMI cups

Two models of the CMI cup are commercially available. The 'Soft Touch' cup is made of malle-able polyethelyne plastic and has a bell-shaped design with flared margins (Fig. 1.13a). It resembles the Mityvac cup very closely in appearance and design. The cup, tubing and fluid trap are available in a pre-packed sterile pouch and are disposable. When the system is used with the CMI vacuum pump, the unit is compact, portable and easy to use. Other benefits claimed for the cup include less scalp marking and injury, fewer de-tachments and more comfort for the mother. The 'Tender Touch' cup was introduced in 1989 (Fig. 1.13b). The cup is manufactured from silicone rubber in the characteristic Kobayashi shape and is reusable after sterilization.

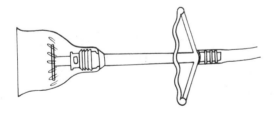

Fig. 1.13(a)   The CMI (tender touch) cup

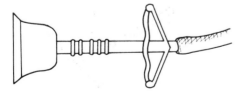

Fig. 1.13(b)   The CMI (soft touch) cup

VACUUM EXTRACTOR CUPS IN COMMON USE

The vacuum extractor cups that are commercially available and in common use are shown in Table 1.1. The Malmstrom and Bird anterior cups are manufactured in three sizes – 40, 50 and 60 mm – whereas the Bird posterior cup is made in one size – 50 mm – and now only as the New Generation type. The O'Neil cups, anterior and posterior, are available in one size, 55 mm. Of the Soft cups, the Silastic and standard Silc cups have internal dia-meters of 65 and 60 mm respectively but a smaller Silc cup of 50 mm is also available. The Mityvac and CMI cups have a diameter of 60 mm across the flared margins of the opening.

Table 1.1   Vacuum extractor cups

Model	Internal diameter (mm)		
Malmstrom	40	50	60
Bird (original)			
Anterior cup	40	50	60
Posterior cup		50	
Bird (New Generation)			
Anterior cup	40	50	60
Posterior cup		50	
O'Neil			
Anterior cup		55	
Posterior cup		55	
Silc		50	60
Silastic			65
Mityvac			60
CMI			
Soft Touch			60
Tender Touch			60

DESCRIPTION AND MAINTENANCE OF EQUIPMENT

Malmstrom cup

The Malmstrom cups are made of stainless steel and are available in 40, 50 and 60 mm sizes. In the centre of the dome of each cup, there is a small metal tube 16 mm long to which is attached sili-cone rubber tubing 15–30 cm long according to the wishes of the operator. At the other end, the tube is attached to a crossed traction handle from which a second, longer silicone rubber tube leads to a vacuum bottle and pump which may be either electrically or manually operated. Traction is applied by means of a chain running inside the rubber tube and across the traction handle where it is transfixed by a stop clip (Fig. 1.14). Earlier versions had a traction handle in which the chain was fastened by a pin, the system being closed by means of a screw cap at one end of the handle (Fig. 1.15). At the fetal end, the chain is attached to a flat metal plate which lies in the hollow of the cup, but which has crennelations in its margin so as to prevent it making an airtight seal (Fig. 1.16). When the apparatus is assembled before use, the tubing is attached both to the cup and to the traction handle, and the chain is threaded through the tubing and pulled tight so as to seat the plate snugly in the apex of the cup. The chain is then transfixed with the clip or pin. To the other end of the traction handle is attached the longer piece of silicone

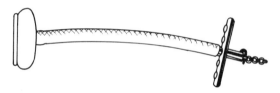

Fig. 1.14 Assembled Malmstrom cup with stop-clip fastener

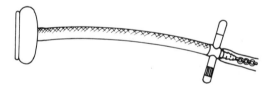

Fig. 1.15 Assembled Malmstrom cup with screw-cap pin fastener

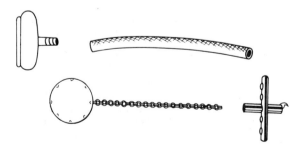

Fig. 1.16 Component parts – metal cup; base plate and traction chain; handle with stop-clip and silicone tube

tubing which may be up to one metre in length and which in turn leads to the vacuum bottle and pump system.

Cleaning, assembling and sterilizing the Malmstrom cup

To separate the Malmstrom device into its component parts, the longer portion of rubber tubing leading from the traction handle to the vacuum bottle is removed and cleaned by running a stream of tap water through it. The traction handle is released by pulling the chain while at the same time holding the handle with the stopclip downwards so that the clip will be released from the link in the chain. The flat stainless steel metal plate inside the cup and the attached chain can then be drawn completely out of the extraction cup. The traction handle may now be removed from the shorter silicone rubber suction tube which in turn can be detached from the extraction cup (Fig. 1.16). All the metal parts may be cleaned with brush, soap and water. The short silicone suction tube can be cleaned by running a stream of tap water through it followed by warm soapy water or alternatively by using a thin, long-handled test tube brush or similar instrument. To reassemble the Malmstrom cup prior to sterilization, the previous steps are performed in reverse order: the shorter silicone rubber tube is pushed on to the tube connector of the vacuum cup; the cup is held with its opening facing upwards in one hand while the other hand holding the metal base plate directs the chain through the hole in the centre of the cup and through the tubing so that the bottom plate fits into place in the apex of the cup. Next, the protruding end of the chain is passed through the tube connector piece of the traction handle which is held in a horizontal position in one hand with the stopclip facing upwards. The chain is grasped with the thumb and forefinger of the other hand and pulled tight. The clip is then allowed to fall into the chain link that is nearest the traction handle tube connector. The cup unit is then reassembled ready for sterilization and subsequent use (see Fig. 1.14). Following reassembly the extraction cup and the long silicone rubber suction tube may be sterilized in the autoclave, preferably in a transparent plastic bag. Sterilization may also be carried out by boiling for 15 minutes. The cup may then be wrapped in a sterile towel ready for use.

Bird cups

The original Bird cups have a chain as the mechanism for traction which is separate from the suction tube. The Anterior cup (Fig. 1.17) has the metal suction pipe eccentrically and obliquely placed on the dome, whereas the Posterior cup (Fig. 1.18) has the pipe attached to the side of the cup. The traction apparatus consists of a welded chain attached permanently to a small, centrally-situated half-ring set into a slight depression on the dome of the cup and a separate handle which can be hooked into an appropriate link of the chain after the cup has been applied to the fetal head. A meshed bottom plate made of polypropylene material is placed within the cup and cannot fall out as its diameter is a little larger than the diameter of the mouth of the cup. Theoretically, the bottom plate functions to maintain a clear space between the fetal scalp and the vacuum tube so that an effective vacuum pressure may be maintained. A short length of silicone rubber tube, approximately 40 cms long is attached to the cup's suction pipe and may be secured against slipping off by a plastic locking ring. The other end of the short tubing is joined through a plastic connector to a longer silicone tube which is attached at its other end to a suitable vacuum pump.

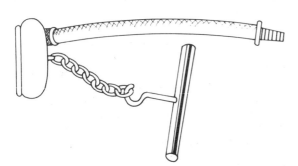

Fig. 1.17   Anterior cup original type

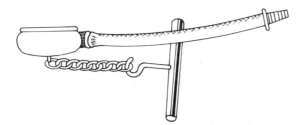

Fig. 1.18   Posterior cup original type

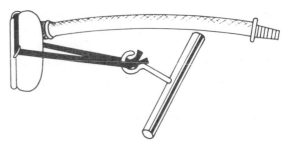

Fig. 1.19   Anterior cup New Generation type

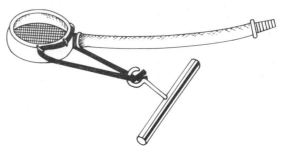

Fig. 1.20   Posterior cup New Generation type

The New Generation Anterior (Fig. 1.19) and Posterior (Fig. 1.20) cups differ from the original models by having a traction cord attached to the rim of the cup by means of welded eyelets around half of the perimeter. In other respects the cups are identical.

Cleaning, assembling and sterilizing the Bird cups

To separate the Bird cups into the component parts (Fig. 1.21), the cup and short length of tubing are disconnected with the plastic connector from the long section of tube. The plastic connector is removed and the short length of tube detached from the cup nozzle and cleaned by running a stream of tap water through it. The polypropylene bottom plate is pulled out of the cup with a finger or with the aid of grasping forceps. All metal parts and the bottom plate are brushed with soap and water. With the New Generation cups, the traction cord knot should be undone, the cord removed and soaked in soapy water and then rinsed in clear water. If satisfactory cleanliness of the cord cannot be achieved, or if the cord is noted to be frayed, it should be replaced with a new one.

To reassemble the cups prior to sterilization, the

polypropylene bottom plate is replaced inside the cup and the short silicone rubber suction tubing is connected to the cup's suction nozzle. If the end of the tube has become soft and does not fit snugly over the metal connecting pipe of the cup, a short piece should be cut from the end of the tube or alternatively a locking ring may be used to secure the tube in order to ensure an airtight seal. For the New Generation cups, the method of attaching the traction cord by threading it through the welded eyelets around half the cup's outer perimeter is shown in Fig. 1.22a. The two ends of the traction cord are brought together and tied in a knot close to the ends of the cord to form a loop which, if the untied cord is supplied in the standard length of 41 cms, should be about 11 cms long (Fig. 1.22b). The reassembled cup and attached short suction tube with universal connector and traction handle

should be packaged in a transparent plastic bag to allow for easy identification and then sterilized by autoclaving. In this form, the cup unit is conveniently available for immediate use. Sterilization of the cups and tubing may also be achieved by boiling.

The O'Neil anterior and posterior cups

The O'Neil cups are supplied as Anterior (Fig. 1.23) and Posterior (Fig. 1.24) models but are manufactured in one size only, 55 mm. The vacuum hose consists of a short piece of silicone tubing fixed to the body of the cup and contains a stainless steel coil which aims to reduce kinking of the tube at its attachment to the cup. A universal connector joins the short piece of tubing to a longer piece from the vacuum pump system. The main difference from the Bird cups is in the traction system. Traction is achieved by means of a looped nylon cord around a curved metal rod attached to the dome of the cup through a rotating base plate.

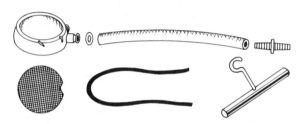

Fig. 1.21 Component parts – posterior new generation cup; optional locking ring; silicone rubber tubing; plastic connector polypropylene bottom plate; nylon traction cord; traction handle

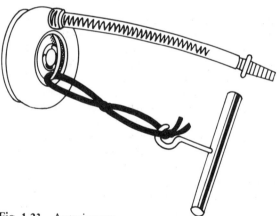

Fig. 1.23 Anterior cup

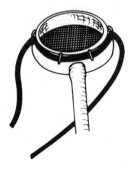

Fig. 1.22(a) Threading the cord

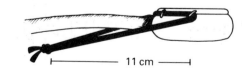

← 11 cm →

Fig. 1.22(b) Tying the cord

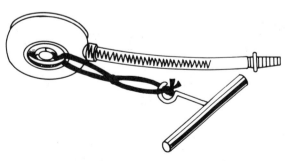

Fig. 1.24 Posterior cup

Cleaning, assembling and sterilizing the O'Neil cups

The polypropylene bottom plate is removed with a finger or forceps and the universal connector is removed from the short piece of tubing. The knot of the traction cord is undone and the cord soaked in soapy water and rinsed with tap water. If satisfactory cleanliness of the cord cannot be achieved, or when the cord is frayed, it should be replaced with a new one. The cup assembly is cleaned with brush and soapy water and the short piece of tube is cleaned by passing a strong jet of tap water through it followed by hot soapy water, using a suitable long handled test tube brush. All parts should then be thoroughly rinsed with tap water.

Before sterilization, the polypropylene bottom plate should be placed in position inside the cup and the protective collar on the end of the short vacuum hose attached to the metal suction tube on the cup body while a universal connector is fitted to the other end of the tubing. A longer piece of tube connects the cup through the connector to a suitable vacuum device. The traction cord is replaced by passing it under the traction collar on the dome of the cup and knotting both ends together so that the cord forms a loop about 11 cms long. A smooth free swivel action of the traction collar should be checked by rotating it fully in both directions. Occasionally it may be necessary to remove the E-clip, traction collar and teflon washers for cleaning (Fig. 1.25). The E-clip may be removed using circlip pliers. To reassemble the traction apparatus, the components are positioned over the stud on the top of the cup in the following order: large washer, traction collar, small washer, E-clip. The reassembled cup and traction handle may be sterilized either by autoclaving, preferably

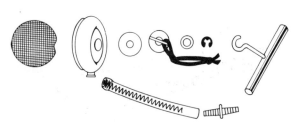

Fig. 1.25 Component parts – polypropylene bottom plate; posterior cup; tubing; universal connector; traction collar with cord attached; teflon washers; E-clip; traction handle

in a transparent plastic packet for easy identification, or by boiling.

The Silastic cup

The Silastic obstetrical vacuum cup (Fig. 1.26) is made from soft silicone material in the shape of a hollow hemisphere and has an inner diameter of 65 mm. A handle through which the suction tube passes is fixed to the dome of the cup, and ridges around the shaft provide a grip for the user. A blue marking line on the cup provides positional reference so that rotation may be observed. The end of the handle is fitted with a chrome-plated brass grip and trumpet valve for vacuum control and release. Projecting beyond the valve is a short metal tube to which is attached a length of suction tube connecting with the vacuum pump. On the inside of the cup there are a number of radial channels spreading out from the central suction tube which allows the air to be evacuated from the space within the cup when it is attached to the fetal head.

Cleaning and sterilizing the Silastic cup

The small vacuum ports and channels on the inside of the cup should be cleaned immediately after use. Fluid and particulate matter should not be allowed to dry and plug these orifices. Sharp instruments, however, should not be used to clean the channels. The cup is cleaned by immersing it in a container of hydrogen peroxide or dilute aqueous solution of acetic acid. The unit is supplied with a blue rubber squeeze bulb to aid in cleaning after use. The bulb is attached to the connector at the end of the handle and the unit is cleansed by flushing the solution in and out. When the channels and ports are cleaned, the cup is washed in mild soap and water and rinsed copiously. It is then wrapped in cloth or placed on a clean open tray and sterilized. With repeat sterilization the cup may become discoloured but this will not affect its physical properties.

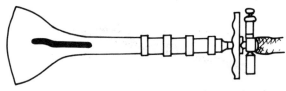

Fig. 1.26 Silastic cup

The Silc cup

The Silc cup (Fig. 1.27) is made of medical grade silicone rubber and is available in two sizes, 50 and 60 mm inner diameter. The instrument is made in one piece and consists of a suction cup and handle. Recently a short version of the cup has been introduced (Fig. 1.28). The cup has a smooth external surface and like the silastic cup is made in the shape of a hollow hemisphere. To the dome of the cup is attached a handle through which passes the suction tube. At the base of the handle, there is a small longitudinal ridge which makes it possible to observe rotation. At the end of the handle, a short metal pipe projects to which is attached a length of tubing that connects the cup to the vacuum apparatus. The inside of the cup is lined with small projections, 1 mm high and 4 mm in diameter, which are separated from one another to allow the air between the cup and the child's head to be evacuated and provide the means of attachment of the cup. The Silc cup is connected to an electric or manual pump by silicone rubber tubing. The partial vacuum recommended for the cup with a 50 mm inner diameter is $0.8 \, \text{kg/cm}^2$ and for the 60 mm cup $0.6 \, \text{kg/cm}^2$. There are no valves in the Silc cup, so increases or decreases of the partial vacuum is achieved by means of a regulator valve on the suction pump.

Cleaning and sterilizing the Silc cup

After use, the cup and tubing should be flushed thoroughly with tap water and washed in soap and water. They are then fitted together, packed and sterilized in a transparent plastic bag following which the instrument is ready for use. Sterilization may be achieved by autoclaving at 120 °C for 20 minutes or by boiling for 15 minutes.

The CMI vacuum cup and delivery system

The Soft Touch CMI vacuum delivery system (Fig. 1.29) consists of a disposable polyethylene plastic cup, tubing and fluid trap which are available in individually pre-packed sterile pouches for use with a pistol-grip hand pump. The cup is bell-shaped with flared margins and an internal diameter of 60 mm with the handle fixed to the top of the cup. On the inside of the cup, there are a number of radial ridges and a fixed plastic base plate. The handle is attached to the dome of the cup and the hollow shaft acts as the suction tube. Near the end of the handle, about 9 cm from the cup, there is a plastic cross bar finger grip. A long piece of plastic tubing is connected to a nozzle at the end of the handle and the other end of the tubing is connected to a fluid trap and through it to the hand pump. The fluid trap is designed to prevent blood or mucus from entering the pump. The pump is hand-operated (Fig. 1.30) and contains a vacuum regulator gauge which is colour

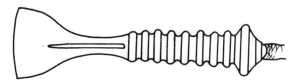

Fig. 1.27   Standard Silc cup

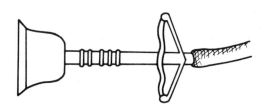

Fig. 1.29(a)   Soft touch CMI cup

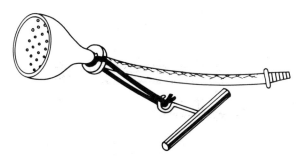

Fig. 1.28   Short Silc cup

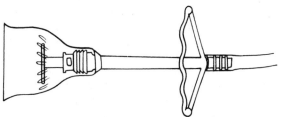

Fig. 1.29(b)   Tender touch CMI cup

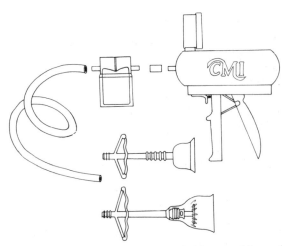

Fig. 1.30 Pistol-grip hand pump; fluid trap; tubing and cup; Soft Touch cup and Tender Touch cup

coded and calibrated both in inches and centimetres of mercury. The pump also incorporates a trigger release valve which allows control of the vacuum pressure. More recently, the reusable CMI Tender Touch cup, a Kobayashi-type silicone instrument, has been introduced. Maintenance is similar to the other silicone cups.

Cleaning and sterilizing the CMI vacuum system

After completing each procedure, the soft touch cup, tubing and fluid trap are discarded. The pump is cleaned with a soft damp cloth which is all that is usually necessary. The trap should prevent fluids from being sucked into the pump during the procedure but if this should happen, the pump should be immediately submerged in clean distilled warm water and the handles squeezed several times to flush out unwanted fluids. The process should be repeated as necessary until the water that is expelled is clear. Fluids should not be allowed to dry inside the pump nor should soap or cleaning solutions be used because they may leave residue which can adversely affect the operation of the pump. When the pump is removed from the water, the handles should be squeezed several times to air dry the internal valves. The CMI vacuum pumps currently being supplied are made of blue plastic material with a stainless steel vacuum gauge (Fig. 1.30). These blue pumps may be autoclaved at 132 °C for 10 minutes. The original white CMI pumps should only be gas sterilized according to the directions from the manufacturer.

VACUUM PUMPS AND SYSTEMS

A number of systems are available for providing the negative pressure required for vacuum extraction and all are satisfactory, provided a control valve is included in the system to regulate the pressure.

Hand and foot pumps

The original pump device consists of a bicycle type hand pump and a glass flask with a pressure gauge in a carrying basket (Fig. 1.31). This system is still widely used. It is supplied with the Malmstrom, Bird and Silc cups, but is suitable for all models. A new version of the portable vacuum hand pump has been developed with changes to the pump and carrying case but the basic components of the system are similar. These small pumps increase the portability and reduce the cost of the apparatus and may be used in circumstances where no electricity supplies are available. However, they require the cooperation of an assistant and, unless maintained in optimum working condition may be difficult to operate.

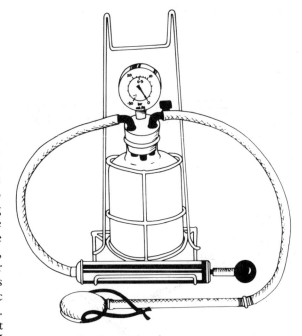

Fig. 1.31 Bicycle-type hand pump vacuum system with regulator valve and pressure gauge, in wire carrying frame

The CMI vacuum system described above (Fig. 1.30) is a lightweight compact hand pump specifically designed for use with the CMI cup but may also be used with other types of cup. The blue coloured pumps may be autoclaved and so can be operated by the obstetrician performing the procedure. In hospitals, reticulated suction has been found to be a suitable source of negative pressure for vacuum extraction provided it is passed through a pressure controlling valve[15] or is connected to the glass bottle of an original vacuum pump device[16]. If reticulated suction is used, regular checks should be made to ensure that the negative pressure is constant and within the working range of the vacuum extractor: 0.6–0.8 kgm/cm^2.

Electric vacuum pumps

Portable electric pumps specifically designed for vacuum extraction are available (Fig. 1.32), and probably are more efficient at forming and maintaining vacuum pressure. The required vacuum pressure may be preset so that, even if leakages occur around the cup or elsewhere in the apparatus, the level will be promptly and automatically restored. Although they are easier to operate, electric pumps have the disadvantage of being heavy and more costly than the simple hand pump systems.

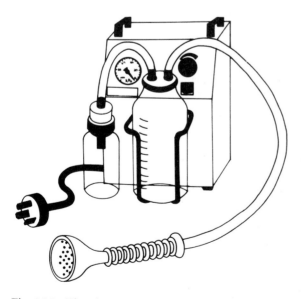

Fig. 1.32 Electric vacuum pump and system

Tubing

Silicone rubber tubing is the preferred type as it does not deteriorate significantly with time or collapse under pressure. Repeat autoclaving, however, may cause softening and stretching at the ends of the tube joining the cup or pump and result in leakage and loss of vacuum. If after trimming a short piece off the ends of the tube the fault is not corrected, the entire length of tubing should be replaced. Locking rings are provided with the Bird cups to prevent such leakage[5], but they are rarely necessary.

An airtight seal within the pump and tubing is crucial to the success of vacuum extraction and cups and pumps should be inspected regularly and maintained in good working order. Electric pumps are efficient and have few maintenance problems but are bulky and more expensive than the hand-held systems. The hand operated devices need to be carefully maintained to ensure reliability but have the advantage of being small in size and comparatively low in cost. Because cleaning and reassembly of the equipment is commonly performed by members of the central sterilizing staff, it is important that they are familiar with the various components of the instrument and know how to maintain the equipment and replace defective parts. A nominated contact person experienced in vacuum extraction should be available for advice and should conduct regular checks of the equipment as a separate procedure from the testing performed by the operator immediately prior to the delivery.

NEGATIVE PRESSURES FOR VACUUM EXTRACTION

The recommended operating vacuum pressures for the majority of the cups are between 0.6 and

Table 1.2 Equivalent negative gauge pressures

Kg/cm$_2$	kPa	mmHg	inches Hg	cm H$_2$O	lb/in^2	bar
0.13	13	100	3.9	134	1.9	0.13
0.27	27	200	7.9	268	3.9	0.26
0.41	40	300	11.8	402	5.8	0.39
0.54	53	400	15.7	536	7.7	0.53
0.68	67	500	19.7	670	9.7	0.66
0.82	80	600	23.6	804	11.6	0.79
0.95	93	700	27.0	938	13.5	0.92
1.03	101	760	29.9	1018	14.7	1.00

0.8 kgm/cm^2. Not all gauges on pumps are standardized to the same units, but easy conversion tables of equivalent negative pressures are available (Table 1.2). The recommendation that up to 10 minutes be allowed to form a chignon before applying traction[3, 17] is unnecessary and the method time consuming. It has been shown that an effective artificial caput succedaneum (chignon) is formed within two minutes of creating a vacuum[18]. Once the operator is satisfied that the cup is applied correctly to the head, the desired vacuum pressure may be achieved in one step and traction commenced after two minutes[19].

Table 1.3 Suppliers of vacuum extraction equipment

Equipment	Address
Malmstrom, Bird, Silc cups (hand and electric pumps)	Menox AB Box 2653 S-40060 GOTHENBURG SWEDEN Telephone: +46 31 802565 Fax: +46 31 196670
O'Neil cups	GO Medical Industries 200 Churchill Avenue SUBIACO WESTERN AUSTRALIA 6008 Telephone: +61 9 3819195 Fax: +61 9 3824952
Silastic cup	Dow Corning Wright P.O. Box 100 ARLINGTON TN 38002 USA Telephone: +1 901 8679971 Fax: +1 901 8674793
CMI cups and handpump	Columbia Medical & Surgical Inc. P.O. Box 5877 BEND OREGON 97708-5877 USA Telephone: +1 503 3880347 Fax: +1 503 3822978
Mityvac cup and handpump	Neward Enterprises Inc. P.O. Box 725 CUCAMONGA CALIFORNIA 91730 USA Telephone: +1 714 987 8975 Fax: +1 714 980 46554
Electric pump	Medela AG Medical Equipment Lattichstrasse 4 6340 BAAR SWITZERLAND Telephone: +41 42 311616 Fax: +41 42 315021

2

CLINICAL PRINCIPLES

GENERAL PRINCIPLES

Progress of the fetus through the birth canal

To progress through the birth canal the fetus must undertake a series of movements that includes descent along a curved pelvic axis with the head undergoing changes of flexion, synclitism, internal rotation and extention. Rydberg[20] described the process as a movement towards a position of least resistance. Mechanical factors that determine movement of the fetal head are:

- the strength and application of the propulsive forces, namely uterine contractions and maternal expulsive effort
- the size, shape and elastic properties of the birth canal
- the size of the fetus
- the shape and weight of the fetal head
- the degree of moulding of the head and size of the caput succedaneum
- the position of the fetal head in the maternal pelvis
- the attitude of the fetal head (flexion or deflexion, synclitism or asynclitism)
- the resistance between fetus and maternal tissue.

While the sizes of the fetus and birth canal are constant, there are a number of factors that influence the progress of labour which are variable and which may be manipulated to reduce resistance between fetus and maternal tissues and make birth easier. Variables such as uterine contractions, maternal expulsive effort, and attitude and position of the fetal head may be altered to improve labour and assist delivery.

The birth canal

The birth canal consists of rigid and soft tissue components and, through dilatation, is transformed into a wide, bent tube displaying elastic properties. Force resulting from contractions acts mainly as a forward drive for the fetal head and this is counterbalanced by the resistance of the soft parts of the birth canal. It is probable that elastic resistance of the soft tissues plays an important role in the production of anterior rotation of the

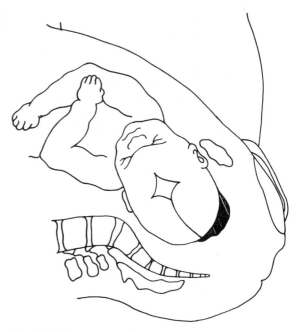

Fig. 2.1 Engagement of the head with anterior asynclitism and the caput succedaneum on the parietal aspect of the head

occiput[20]. The more rigid portions of the birth canal may also impose restrictions on the movements of the fetal head and direct the occiput anteriorly, since the converging sidewalls make it difficult for the head to descend in a transverse and unflexed state for the entire length of the passage. It has been shown that transverse and posterior positions of the head are normal at the pelvic inlet and upper regions of the birth canal[21] and that when engagement of the head occurs the sagittal suture is usually situated behind the transverse diameter of the pelvic cavity, closer to the sacrum (Fig. 2.1). This degree of anterior asynclitism is common in normal labour and occurs because of the posterior inclination of the axis of the pelvis at these levels. It also causes the parietal aspect of the fetal head to become the presenting part and explains why the caput succedaneum forms often on the parietal region when delay in labour occurs and the position of the occiput is lateral or posterior.

Shape of the fetal head

The fetal head is commonly described as ovoid in shape (Fig. 2.2) with the mentovertical diameter exceeding all others in length[22] but Rydberg described the head as a kidney-shaped body having its convexity upwards and forwards with the greater volume of the head lying above and in front of the mentovertical plane[20]. He showed that if an oval body like the fetal head is pushed through a curved canal with an elastic wall, it will generally turn in such a way that one pole precedes and deviates in the direction of the canal, provided the

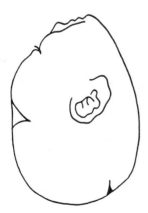

Fig. 2.2 Shape of the head

dimensions of the canal are too narrow to allow the body to fall through it in any position.

Mechanical energy derived from uterine contractions is used to mould the fetal head and to dilate the soft tissues of the birth canal. Provided the volume of amniotic fluid is adequate, pressure within the uterus is distributed evenly throughout the cavity but is not necessarily equal on all parts of the fetal head[23]. The pressure during normal labour at the largest circumference of the head has been calculated to be three to four times greater than the corresponding amniotic pressure and tone. Above and below the largest diameters, the measured pressures were found to be less than the maximum. Since force at the largest circumference of the fetal head operates mainly at right angles to the pelvic axis and is greater than the pressure along the axis, the fetal head becomes elongated or moulded. Prolonged labour with the occiput lateral or posterior may produce excessive moulding of the head and cause a large parietal caput succedaneum to form. These changes alter the shape of the head and may prevent or interfere with normal internal rotational movements[20].

Diameters of the head in vertex presentations

Attitude and position of the fetal head in the pelvis will cause the size of the area of the presenting part to vary and thus may influence the progress of labour in circumstances where the relationship between the size of the fetus and the maternal pelvis is borderline. Optimum presenting diameters of the head within the birth canal, the sub-occipitobregmatic and biparietal[22] occur when the head is completely flexed and synclitic (Fig. 2.3). When the fetal head is flexed but asynclitic, the sub-occipitobregmatic diameter may be unchanged but the width of the oblique biparietal diameter is increased (Fig. 2.4). Deflexion of the head causes a lengthening of the sagittal diameter starting from the suboccipitobregmatic to occipitofrontal (Fig. 2.5) and in extreme cases to the mentovertical diameter of a brow presentation. If asynclitism is present as well as deflexion, lengthening will occur in all the diameters in the sagittal (occipitofrontal) and coronal (biparietal) planes (Fig. 2.6). Although the usual outcome with such presentations is for further flexion and synclitism to occur during descent with subsequent anterior rotation of the occiput, progress may become arrested if these changes do not take place.

PRESENTING DIAMETERS OF THE VERTEX

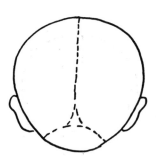

Fig. 2.3 Flexion and synclitism

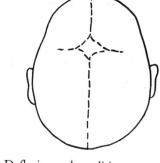

Fig. 2.5 Deflexion and synclitism

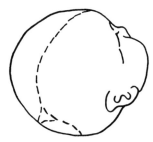

Fig. 2.4 Flexion and asynclitism

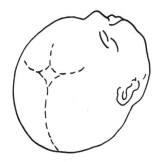

Fig. 2.6 Deflexion and asynclitism

Some form of intervention may then become necessary to assist the mother to give birth.

The flexion point

Positional flexion of the head develops to some extent before the onset of labour and occurs most likely as a result of the shape of the head and its relationship to the birth canal. Complete flexion of the head exists when the mentovertical diameter points in the direction of the pelvic axis[20]. In a normally moulded fetal head, the mentovertical diameter emerges on the sagittal suture approximately 3 cms in front of the posterior fontanelle (Fig. 2.7). This 'flexion point' is an important landmark for vacuum extraction.

TECHNICAL PRINCIPLES

Position of the vacuum cup

Correct technique with the vacuum extractor should enhance the normal process of labour and should not depend on traction alone to effect delivery of the baby[3]. When a vacuum cup is attached to the head and traction is applied, the cup becomes the leading part provided there is room enough in the birth canal for the head to move[9]. For this reason the centre of the cup should correspond as closely as possible to the flexion point so that traction in the line of the pelvic axis will promote flexion and synclitism and result in the most favourable presenting diameters (Fig. 2.8). In practice, therefore, ideal application of the vacuum cup is achieved when the centre of the cup is superimposed on the flexion point and the cup is symmetrically placed over the sagittal suture. This

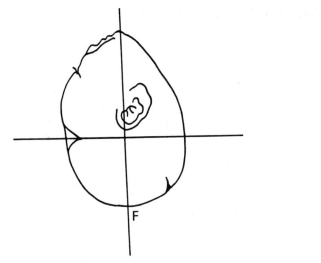
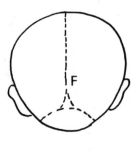

Fig. 2.7   The flexion point (F)

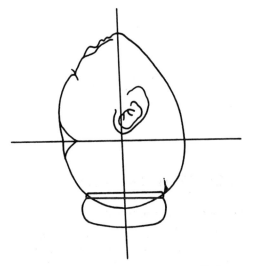
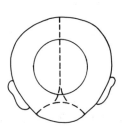
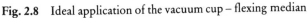
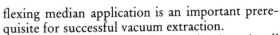

Fig. 2.8   Ideal application of the vacuum cup – flexing median

flexing median application is an important prerequisite for successful vacuum extraction.

To achieve flexing median applications in all positions of the occiput, some basic knowledge of the sizes of vacuum cups in relation to the dimensions of the vertex may be helpful. Each cup receives its nominal size from the internal diameter across the opening but, because many of the cups have curved sides, the diameter through the body of the cup may be greater[24]. For example, a metal cup with a diameter of 50 mm across the opening

has a maximum diameter of 60 mm. The external diameters of the vacuum extractor cups in common use range from 50–70 mm. Because the posterior fontanelle is obscured and may be difficult or impossible to identify when the cup is correctly placed on the fetal head, the anterior fontanelle should be used as the main positional reference point. It should also be appreciated that the distance between anterior and posterior fontanelles in the newborn infant at term is approximately 9 cms so that, by extrapolation, the flexion point will be located on the sagittal suture 6 cms behind the anterior fontanelle (Fig. 2.9). Thus, when the centre of a 50 mm cup is placed over the flexion point, the posterior 6 cms of the sagittal suture line will be covered by the cup, leaving 3 cms at the anterior end exposed. This distance between the leading edge of the cup and the anterior fontanelle has been called the application distance[9]. In practice, the operator can confirm that the cup is correctly positioned when a space of 3 cms or more can be palpated between the anterior fontanelle and the nearest part of the cup and when the sagittal suture passes under the centre of the cup[25].

If the centre of the cup is situated more than 1 cm to either side of the sagittal suture, the application is described as paramedian; and when the application distance is less than 3 cms it is called deflexing. Thus there are four types of cup applications (Fig. 2.10): (a) flexing median; (b) flexing paramedian, (c) deflexing median and (d) deflexing paramedian. Deflexing and paramedian

applications promote extension and asyncliticism of the head and effectively increase or fail to decrease the size of the area of the presenting part (Figs 2.11, 2.12 and 2.13).

In an observational study of 389 consecutive vacuum extractions[26] performed by operators at all levels of experience, correct (flexing median) applications were recorded in just over half of the procedures (Fig. 2.14). Analysis of application sites according to positions of the head when the cup was applied revealed that fewer correct applications were achieved in occipitolateral and occipitoposterior positions. Indeed, when the occiput was posterior, 70 per cent of the applications were either deflexing, paramedian or both. Failure rates for each type of application were: flexing median 4 per cent; flexing paramedian 17 per cent; deflexing median 29 per cent; and deflexing paramedian 35 per cent. Such findings support the view that difficult and failed vacuum extractions and subsequent caesarean section for disproportion are sometimes the result of cup applications that promote or fail to correct deflexion and asynclitism[9].

Location of the flexion point

In order to achieve flexing median applications in all positions of the occiput, the operator must know the location of the flexion point and be able to place the centre of the cup precisely over that point. The flexion point may be located during vaginal examination by identifying the posterior fontanelle and then moving the finger anteriorly a distance of approximately 3 cms along the sagittal suture. The tip of the finger will mark the flexion point.

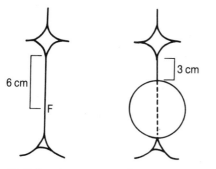

Fig. 2.9 Defining the correct application of the vacuum cup over the flexion point (F)

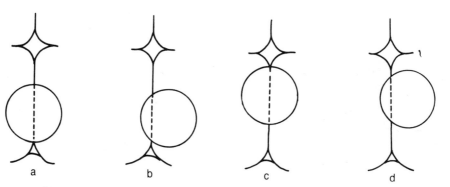

Fig. 2.10 Correct and incorrect applications:
(a) flexing median; (b) flexing paramedian; (c) deflexing median; (d) deflexing paramedian

DIAMETERS OF THE PRESENTING PART RELATED TO CUP APPLICATION

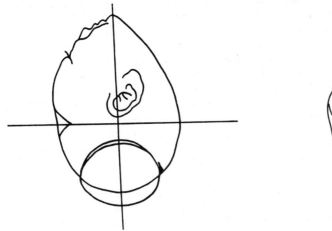
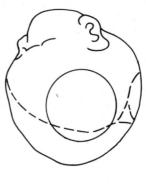

Fig. 2.11 Flexing paramedian

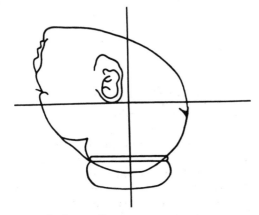
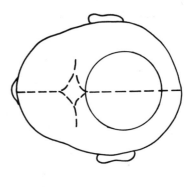

Fig. 2.12 Deflexing median

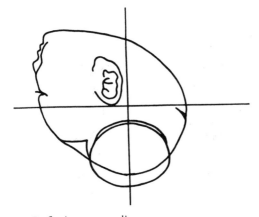
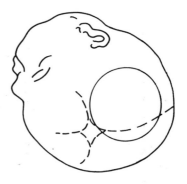

Fig. 2.13 Deflexing paramedian

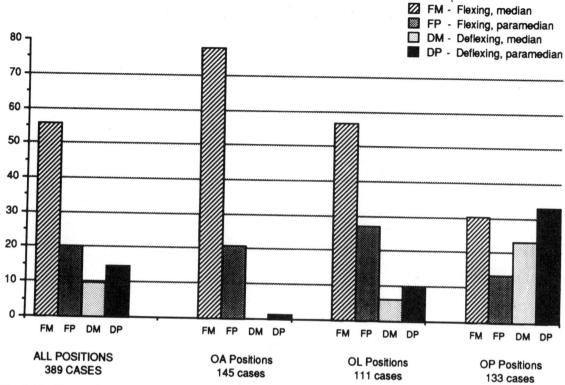

Fig. 2.14 Types of application of the cup related to position of the head

The flexion point will be situated in the centre of the introitus and within the presenting part when the sagittal suture is vertical and the fetal head is completely flexed. These conditions apply when the head is visible at the outlet of the pelvis and also on most occasions when it has descended to the level of the pelvic floor (Fig. 2.15). Attaching the vacuum cup to the most accessible portion of the presenting part in these circumstances will achieve a flexing median application. Sometimes, however, when the head is on the pelvic floor, the sagittal suture may be situated in the right or left oblique position and a slight degree of asynclitism may be present. The flexion point will not be in the centre of the introitus but displaced to one side (Fig. 2.16) and, unless the cup is manoeuvred laterally, the resulting application will be flexing, but (most likely) paramedian.

In mid-cavity occipitolateral positions, the flexion point is often behind (i.e. more sacral) the leading part of the head (Fig. 2.17). This may be a normal finding during labour, due to the direction of the pelvic axis, but if the labour is complicated by deep transverse arrest, the displacement of the flexion point may be exaggerated due to anterior asynclitism. In these lateral positions of the occiput, application of the vacuum cup to the most accessible part of the head without careful localization of the flexion point will frequently result in paramedian applications because the parietal aspect of the head is the presenting part.

If the fetal head is not completely flexed, the application may also be deflexing. Deflexing and paramedian applications of the cup are common in mid pelvic occipitoposterior positions because the flexion point is frequently situated behind the leading part of the head and there is usually some degree of extension and asynclitism associated with these positions (Fig. 2.18). The technique of localizing the flexion point is described in Chapter 5 (see p. 43).

Manoeuvrability of vacuum cups

For a vacuum cup to be applied correctly to the fetal head, the flexion point must lie within the

THE LOCATION OF THE FLEXION POINT

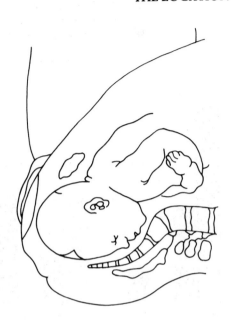

Fig. 2.15　Direct occipitoanterior position

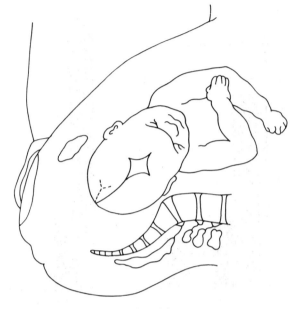

Fig. 2.17　Occipitolateral position

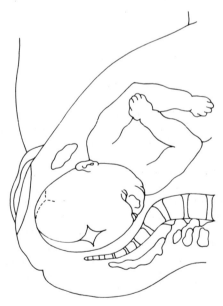

Fig. 2.16　Oblique occipitoanterior position

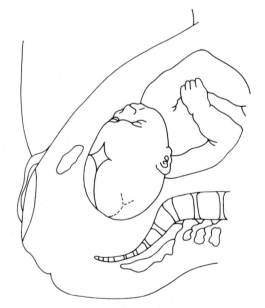

Fig. 2.18　Occipitoposterior position

range of lateral movement of the cup. Examination of the position of the chignon (cup caput) after delivery shows that the cup often fails to reach the ideal application site especially when the occiput is posterior or lateral. Correct application of the vacuum cup depends on:

- knowledge of the location of the flexion point and of the methods of applying the cup in all positions of the occiput
- the experience of the operator with the vacuum extractor and familiarity with the type of cup that is used
- the level of the fetal head
- the position of the occiput
- the extent of deflexion and asynclitism
- the manoeuvrability of the cup.

Manoeuvrability of the vacuum cup within the birth canal depends on:

- the elastic resistance of the tissues of the vulva and perineum
- the available space between head and maternal pelvis
- the size of the caput succedaneum
- the depth and diameter of the cup
- the design of the cup with regard to the position and pliability of the suction tube.

Manoeuvrability of cups with dome-attached suction tubing or handles is limited by the tube pressing against the labial tissues and perineum. The extent of the lateral movement will then be restricted by the elastic resistance of the tissues of the vulva. The Soft cups (Silastic, Silc and CMI) are manoeuvred by pushing the cups in the direction of the flexion point until further movement is

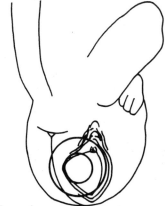

Fig. 2.19 Lateral movement of Soft cups is restricted by vulval tissues

prevented (Fig. 2.19). These cups are suitable for occipitoanterior and well flexed occipitolateral positions where the flexion point is near the introitus (Fig. 2.20a, b, c). They are not suitable for use in the majority of midcavity occipitoposterior or deflexed occipitolateral positions because the flexion point in these cases is usually located outside the range of movement of the cups making it difficult or impossible to achieve a correct application (Fig. 2.21 a, b, c).

The Malmstrom and Anterior cups are generally smaller and shallower than the Soft cups and in theory should be more manoeuvrable. As with the Soft cups, however, lateral movement of these cups is constrained by the tissues of the perineum and vulva making them suitable for anterior positions of the occiput (Fig. 2.22, a and b) but less useful in malpositions (Fig. 2.23, a and b). Bird[4] claimed that the eccentric oblique suction tube of the Anterior cup did not obstruct the process of application as much as cups such as the Malmstrom or the Soft models with a central vertical tube. The centre of the Anterior cup may be moved closer to the flexion point not only by direct movement but also by rotating the cup towards the flexion point using the tube attachment as the pivot point (Fig. 2.24). Although there may be advantages with the anterior design when the position of the head is obliquely anterior, the benefits are not great when the occiput is lateral or posterior.

The Posterior cup is not restricted in its movements by the soft tissues of the vulva and perineum because the suction tube is in the same plane as the body of the cup (Fig. 2.25). This feature allows the cup to be easily inserted through the introitus, manoeuvred under the caput and be directed towards and over the flexion point. Movement of the cup in the birth canal is limited only by the amount of space between the fetal head and mother's sacrum posteriorly and the side walls of the pelvis laterally. Provided the operator is skilled in the use of this cup, flexing median applications may be achieved consistently in nearly all malpositions of the occiput. More manoeuvrable cups should, by permitting better applications, decrease failure rate when the occiput is lateral or obliquely posterior.

Traction

The axis of the pelvis is an imaginary line representing the path followed by the midpoint of the

MANOEUVRABILITY OF THE SOFT CUPS

IN OCCIPITOANTERIOR POSITIONS

IN OCCIPITOPOSTERIOR POSITIONS

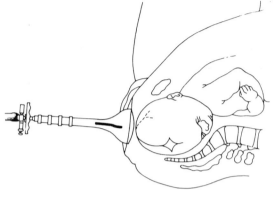

Fig. 2.20(a)

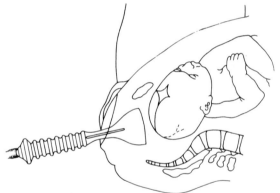

Fig. 2.21(a)

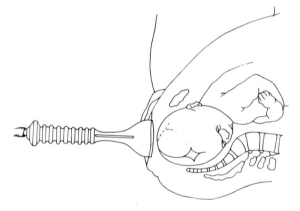

Fig. 2.20(b)

Fig. 2.21(b)

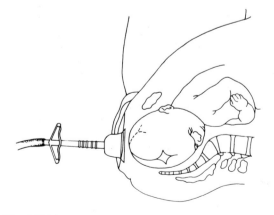

Fig. 2.20(c)

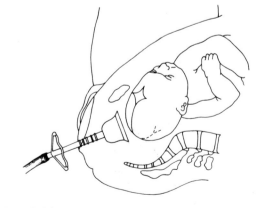

Fig. 2.21(c)

MANOEUVRABILITY OF MALMSTROM AND ANTERIOR CUPS

IN OCCIPITOANTERIOR POSITIONS

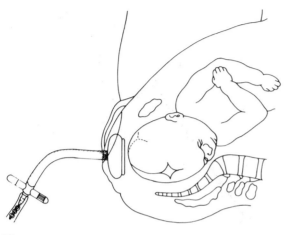

Fig. 2.22(a)

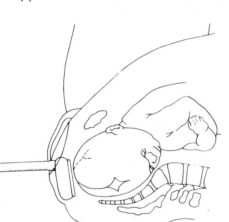

Fig. 2.22(b)

IN OCCIPITOPOSTERIOR POSITIONS

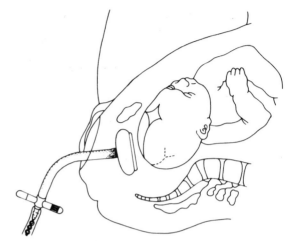

Fig. 2.23(a)

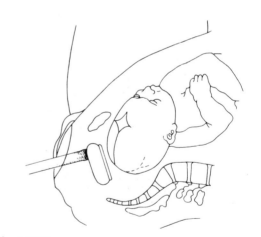

Fig. 2.23(b)

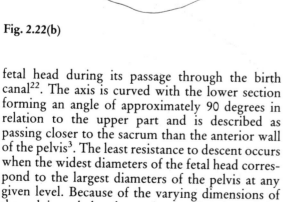

fetal head during its passage through the birth canal[22]. The axis is curved with the lower section forming an angle of approximately 90 degrees in relation to the upper part and is described as passing closer to the sacrum than the anterior wall of the pelvis[3]. The least resistance to descent occurs when the widest diameters of the fetal head correspond to the largest diameters of the pelvis at any given level. Because of the varying dimensions of the pelvis and the change in the direction of the

axis, the fetal head adopts the most favourable position by undertaking a series of movements that includes flexion, synclitism and rotation. For practical purposes, the smallest diameters of the head will be presenting when the mentovertical diameter or its lowermost point, the flexion point, coincides with the direction of the pelvic axis. Operators should realize that this may not be strictly correct because the midpoint of the head is located at the bifurcation of the mentovertical and

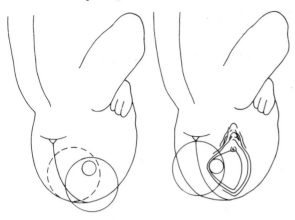

Fig. 2.24 Enhancing the manoeuvrability of the anterior cup

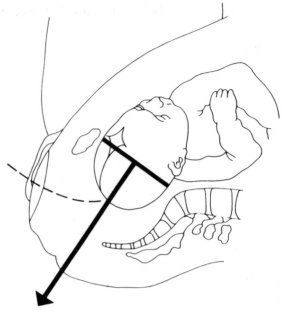

Fig. 2.26 Axis traction for mid pelvic stations (M = midpoint of the head)

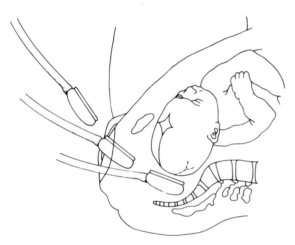

Fig. 2.25 Movement is not impeded by the soft tissues of the birth canal because the body of the cup and suction tube are in the same plane

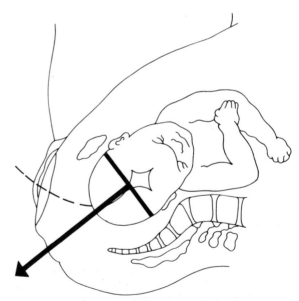

Fig. 2.27 Axis traction for low mid stations

biparietal diameters, some 5 or 6 cms from the flexion point (Fig. 2.26). For this reason, traction should be directed more posteriorly to achieve the best fit of the head within the cavity of the pelvis at any given level. With the mother placed in the lithotomy position and when the level of the fetal head is mid pelvic, the mentovertical diameter will be pointing in a downward direction (towards the floor). The direction of traction therefore for the initial pull should be directed downwards in order to achieve axis traction. The extent to which axis traction is possible will depend on how far the perineum will stretch in that direction. If satisfac-

tory axis traction cannot be achieved, episiotomy may allow traction in a more correct direction by straightening out the lower part of the birth canal. As the head descends to the low-mid level of the

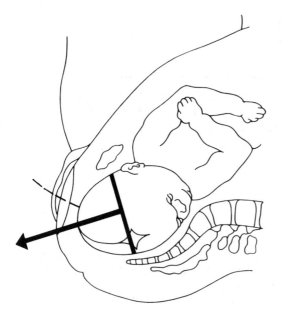

Fig. 2.28 Axis traction for pelvic floor stations

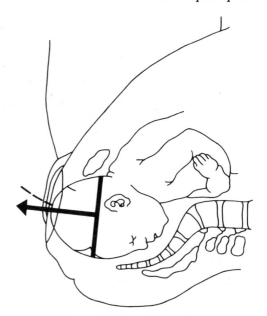

Fig. 2.29 Axis traction for outlet stations

pelvis, the direction to achieve axis traction will not need to be angled so acutely downwards (Fig. 2.27). With further descent and correction of deflexion and asynclitism, the cup becomes visible within the vagina. The operator must resist the tendency to change direction of traction too soon because the axis of the fetal head at the level of the midpoint requires that traction should continue to be directed more posteriorly. When the head descends to the level of the pelvic floor (Fig. 2.28),

the cup will be visible at the outlet and the operator should direct traction horizontally or even slightly downwards in order to keep the axis of the fetal head pointing in the correct line. Once the head has descended to the outlet of the pelvis and the sagittal suture is directly anteroposterior, traction should be directed progressively upwards until the head has crowned and then delivered (Fig. 2.29). Traction technique is described in Chapter 5.

3

SELECTION OF PATIENTS FOR VACUUM EXTRACTION

INDICATIONS AND CONTRAINDICATIONS

There are marked regional and international variations in almost every aspect of operative delivery in obstetric practice[27]: in the rates of total operative delivery; in the relative proportions of instrumental, vaginal and caesarean delivery; in the choice of forceps or vacuum extraction; and in the rates of change in all of these over time[28]. The reasons for such wide variations are not altogether clear but in some cases they reflect differences in obstetrical characteristics and attitudes of the population being served[29], and also may vary with the definition of need for instrumental delivery as perceived by individual practitioners[30]. There is little doubt that the vacuum extractor may cause injury to the mother or baby when the basic ground rules for its use are contravened. As interventions are applied to an increasingly large proportion of the obstetric and fetal population, a threshold will inevitably be reached beyond which the marginal risks of the procedure will outweigh the marginal benefits[30]. The experience of the operator and the selection of cases suitable for instrumental delivery are critical elements in determining whether the benefits of intervention will outweigh the risks. Active management of labour[31] and extension of the limits for the duration of the second stage – provided fetal distress is not present – are measures that may be used to reduce the number of operative deliveries. However, when all other measures fail, there will be a group of patients in whom the choice of delivery will lie between caesarean section and instrumental delivery. In this group, it is essential to recognize the obstetric conditions associated with risk to the fetus and mother and to select the most appropriate method of delivery, taking into consideration the skill and experience of the operator.

Vacuum extraction should not be attempted if cephalopelvic disproportion is present[32], or when the station of the fetal head is high[33]. The practice of applying the cup to a head in order to bring down the presenting part to a lower station so that delivery may be completed with forceps should be discouraged. The vacuum extractor is not suitable for face presentation, nor for delivery of the after coming head in breech presentation. Most brow presentations are contraindications, unless the operator is able to achieve an application of the cup that results in flexion of the head[33]. Although vacuum extraction has been employed successfully to assist birth in preterm infants[2], forceps delivery is generally recommended if the gestation is less than 36 weeks[25, 34]. Vacuum extraction before the cervix is fully dilated may be hazardous for the fetus and mother[35] and should not be attempted unless strict criteria have been satisfied[25], nor should the instrument be used in circumstances associated with significant reduction in maternal expulsive powers such as general anaesthesia[36]. Haemorrhage from the scalp and formation of cephalhaematoma have been described with vacuum extraction following the use of scalp electrodes and after fetal blood sampling[37], but these complications were not encountered in other series[38, 39, 40] and such procedures should not be regarded as contraindications.

Although few medical indications for vacuum extraction are constant and not easily fitted into tidy self-contained categories[28], it is advisable to

Table 3.1 Standard and special indications

Standard (lower risk) indications	Special (higher risk) indications
(*The fetal head is engaged and the cervix is fully dilated.*)	Delay in the second stage associated with fetal malposition and suspected borderline disproportion
Delay in the second stage with the fetal head stationed at the outlet; on the pelvic floor; in the mid pelvis	Acute fetal distress
Subacute fetal distress	Delay or fetal distress associated with fetal malposition in a multipara after the cervix is widely but not fully dilated
Elective shortening of the second stage for fetal or maternal benefit	Delivery of the second twin when the head is not quite engaged or the cervix not completely dilated
	Prolapse of the umbilical cord when the cervix is fully dilated and the head is deeply engaged
	After symphysiotomy

separate them broadly into standard (lower risk) and special (higher risk) groups (Table 3.1). The special uses of the vacuum extractor will be contraindications for all but the most experienced operators. Even when a clear cut indication for expediting birth of the baby exists, a number of other factors which may influence the outcome must be considered before vacuum extraction is attempted. These include dilatation of the cervix; condition of the fetus and mother, uterine contractions; progress in the first stage of labour; duration of the second stage; station, position and moulding; recognition of cephalopelvic disproportion; and experience of the operator.

Dilatation of the cervix

Caution has been advised when using the vacuum extractor before the cervix is fully dilated[25, 32], although there are a number of reports documenting its use in these circumstances[24, 29, 41, 42]. Such procedures should never be attempted by inexperienced or occasional operators because they are generally more complicated and more likely to result in injury to the fetus and mother[35]. The

difficulty arises because the presenting part is usually stationed in the mid pelvis or higher, the occiput is frequently lateral or posterior and the incompletely dilated cervix often hinders correct application of the cup over the ideal site or may be sucked under the cup when the vacuum is induced. In societies where caesarean section is regarded to be a hazardous and culturally unacceptable procedure for the mother, vacuum extraction in the first stage of labour may be considered to be the safer alternative[29] but, in most circumstances, caesarean section should be the preferred method of delivery. A few exceptions to this rule may be permissible, provided the operator has been adequately trained and cephalopelvic disproportion has been confidently excluded[25]; to assist the birth of the second twin and for correcting malposition in a multipara whose cervix is almost fully dilated. In general, however, unless these specific criteria apply, delivery should be completed by caesarean section.

Condition of the fetus and mother

If it is decided to assist the birth with the vacuum extractor, the attendant should explain the reasons for the procedure to the mother and emphasize the need for her cooperation and active involvement. The greater the maternal expulsive effort, the less traction effort will be needed to assist the delivery. The mother's ability to push effectively will depend to some extent on her physical and emotional state. Physical exhaustion may occur at any stage during active labour but is more likely during the expulsive phase of the second stage when the extra effort of pushing is added to the stress of contractions[43]. Even if the mother is not physically distressed, her morale and emotional state may influence the extent to which she will become involved in the birth. An unsatisfactory maternal experience of childbirth has been associated most clearly with prolonged labour resulting in forceps delivery and not so much with pain[44]. Fetal distress and delay in the second stage of labour are common indications for instrumental delivery and under these circumstances it is hardly surprising that maternal anxiety is increased. Some of that anxiety may be relieved if the mother and her partner are fully informed of the reasons for operative delivery and if they receive continuous support[39].

In medical conditions where excessive maternal

exertion is contraindicated during the expulsion phase, forceps are usually preferred since they are less dependant on maternal effort. However, the vacuum extractor may be employed in such situations if the fetal head is allowed time to descend to the pelvic floor, using oxytocin infusion if necessary to maintain normal uterine action, and epidural analgesia to reduce any urge to push prematurely[41]. Steady traction synchronous with contractions and an application of the vacuum cup that promotes flexion of the head will nearly always result in easy delivery without undue effort on the part of the mother. The vacuum extractor is sometimes regarded to be too slow for use in severe fetal distress but in experienced hands the application-to-delivery interval need be no longer for vacuum extraction than for forceps[39]. If the operator is inexperienced or if difficulty is anticipated, an alternative method of delivery – either forceps or caesarean section – may be preferable. A normal fetal blood pH estimation may be of assistance in allowing labour to continue until spontaneous delivery occurs or the head descends to a lower station, making vacuum extraction easier.

Uterine contractions

Studies of uterine activity in labour indicate that the uterus generates whatever activity is necessary to expel the fetus within the biological restraint imposed on it[45]. The uterus increases its efforts to a maximum depending on the degree of resistance it meets, after which the efficiency usually decreases, resulting in lower uterine activity. Hypotonic uterine action is more common in the primigravid uterus and may occur in the first and second stage of labour[46]. In the nulliparous patient with inefficient uterine action, and a healthy fetus, contractions should be stimulated with oxytocin to mimic the normal pattern. On the other hand, in the multiparous woman, inefficient uterine action is less common and caution is required before introducing oxytocin to increase uterine activity because of the risks of hypertonic contractions and rupture of the uterus. Careful assessment should be made by an experienced obstetrician to exclude disproportion before administering oxytocin for delay in the first or second stage of labour. Abdominal palpation cannot accurately measure the intensity of uterine contractions and this constraint also applies to the record made by an external tocodynamometer. Intrauterine pressure recording may enable better evaluation of the progress of labour and provide a means of monitoring changes in uterine activity in response to treatment with oxytocin but these methods are not always available, nor have the postulated benefits been demonstrated by controlled clinical trials[47].

Successful vacuum extraction depends on effective uterine contractions and maternal expulsive effort. Malmstrom emphasized the importance of establishing cooperation with the expulsive forces generated by the uterus[23]. He also pointed out that continuous weak traction with the vacuum extractor may improve uterine contractions as a result of the head pressing on the lower uterine segment and cervix[3, 32], but oxytocin by infusion is a more reliable and safer method[24, 34, 36]. Oxytocin introduced at the onset of the second stage of labour has been shown to shorten the duration of the second stage[48]. There was also an increase in spontaneous deliveries and a decrease in the overall numbers of instrumental procedures but the number of rotational forceps was unchanged in the oxytocin group. Once the decision has been made to assist delivery by vacuum extraction, the operator should have no hesitation in introducing oxytocin to enhance contractions.

Progress in the first stage of labour

Prolonged labour may result in physical and emotional exhaustion of the mother as well as perinatal asphyxia of the fetus[47]. Should vacuum extraction be required to assist the delivery, the procedure may be more hazardous for the baby if maternal participation is reduced through exhaustion. For these reasons, the prevention or early detection of prolonged labour should be a major objective of all birth attendants. Poor progress in labour is most commonly due to ineffective uterine action, a condition which nearly always responds to augmentation with oxytocin[31].

Assessment of progress and recognition of prolonged labour depends on knowing the time of onset of the labour but this information may not always be clear from the mother's history and examination. For this reason, the time of admission to the delivery room is the most practical reference point marking the start of supervised labour, and the rate of cervical dilatation is the most useful means of assessing progress. Because there may be considerable interobserver variation

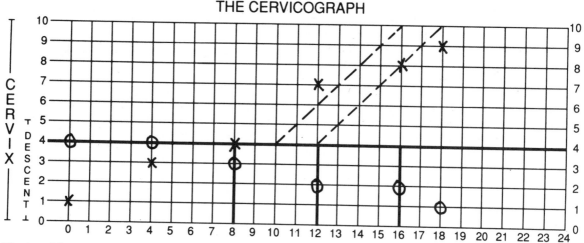

Fig. 3.1 The cervicograph crossing the warning and action lines; X = Cervical dilatation, O = level of the head (After Bird, 1978)

in estimates of cervical dilatation, vaginal examination should be performed or confirmed by an experienced birth attendant. The dilatation should be assessed between contractions taking care not to stretch the cervix when performing the examination. Dilatation should be recorded in whole centimetres; if the estimate should fall between two numbers, the more conservative value should be taken. This may be of considerable importance if cervical dilatation is the observation used to differentiate latent from active phase of labour.

Although initial cervimetric studies concentrated on labours of nulliparous women, the rate of cervical dilatation in the active phase of spontaneous labour has been found to be similar in multigravidae and that it was not affected by racial differences[49, 50]. Philpott and Castle[51] devised a practical method of distinguishing normal from abnormal progress in labour by plotting cervical dilatation against time on graph paper (the cervicograph) and relating it to 1 cm/hour reference lines which they called 'alert' and 'action' lines. The alert line corresponded roughly to the mean rate of cervical dilatation in the slowest 10 per cent of the primigravidae in their study but when the cervicograph was introduced into routine obstetric practice it was found that the line was crossed by more than 20 per cent of the women. With too narrow a definition of normality, there is the risk that an increased number of labours will be incorrectly defined as abnormal and that the women concerned might be subjected to unnecessary interventions to treat non-existent dystocia[48]. Bird[53]

suggested that a reduction in the number of women whose cervicographs incorrectly identified abnormal progress in labour (false positives) could be achieved by modifying the original definition of the onset of the active phase of labour on the cervicograph from 3–4 cm and also by moving the position of the alert line two hours to the right (Fig. 3.1). He also stressed the importance of not overestimating dilatation of the cervix when the reference lines were drawn and described the procedure to be followed when the action line was crossed. The visual impact of the graph crossing the action line allows the medical and midwifery attendant to recognize abnormal progress in labour early and to institute appropriate management. The cervicograph has been incorporated into a composite labour record, the partogram, which displays the condition of the fetus and mother as well as progress in labour on a single sheet of paper[54].

Duration of the second stage

Although the precise onset and actual length of the second stage of labour is usually not known, the normal duration has been traditionally stated to be somewhere between 1 and 2 hours for a nulliparous woman and between 30 minutes and 1 hour for a multipara[55, 56]. Studies have shown an association between prolonged second stage of labour and infant mortality, increased incidence of early neonatal seizures and poor perinatal and long term outcome. However, when these studies were subjected to logistic regression analysis to allow for possible confounding influences, prolonged duration of the second stage on its own was shown to be of little significance[54]. For this reason, it has been suggested that prolongation of the second stage of labour should not be regarded as a reason in itself for intervention provided the mother and baby's condition is satisfactory and there is a progressive descent of the presenting part.

For the purposes of management it may be helpful to divide the second stage of labour into two distinct phases[56]. The first phase extends from the time of full dilatation of the cervix until the fetal head reaches the pelvic floor and may be regarded as an extension of the first stage of labour. The second phase extends from the time the head reaches the pelvic floor until the baby is born. Liberal use of oxytocin may be better than premature instrumental delivery for the treatment of delay in the first phase of the second stage of labour. Such an approach, combined with a policy of active management of labour based on the provision of effective uterine contractions in the first stage, resulted in a marked reduction in the incidence of abnormal labours due to occipitoposterior position and a corresponding reduction in the number of midcavity forceps procedures[57].

Although a more conservative approach to delay in the second stage of labour may result in some babies who might otherwise have had instrumental deliveries being born spontaneously, those who do require assistance may form a higher risk group for vacuum extraction because the obstetric conditions in this group may be less favourable for instrumental delivery. For example, uterine action may be less effective after prolonged labour and physical discomfort or exhaustion may reduce the contribution of the mother's expulsive effort to the birth. Furthermore, a prominent caput succedaneum and advanced moulding of the head are likely to be present when the duration of the second stage is prolonged, and this combination of factors may confuse the diagnosis of position and station of the head. Increasing moulding and the presence of a large caput may also mislead the examiner into thinking that the presenting part has descended, when in fact it has undergone a change of shape. For these reasons, when the second stage is prolonged, assessment of the condition of the fetus and mother, rate of progress of labour and suitability for vacuum extraction may require considerable obstetric judgement and should be per-

formed only by experienced attendants.

Station, position and moulding of the fetal head

Station of the head

Station may be assessed by relating the lowermost portion of the presenting part to the ischial spines. By this method, engagement of the head has been defined as having occurred when the presenting part is at or below the ischial spines, for at this stage the biparietal diameter of the head is assumed to have passed through the plane of the brim of the pelvis. In normal labours, such an assumption is usually correct but in difficult situations where pronounced moulding causes elongation of the head, or where a prominent caput succedaneum obscures a clear definition of the lowest cranial point, the head may appear to be lower in the pelvis than is actually the case[26]. When the presenting part is at the level of the ischial spines, it is designated as being at zero station. If the head is above the spines, the station is given a minus value and, if it is below the spines, a plus value. Care must be taken not to overestimate descent of the head because adverse outcomes are more likely with mid or high pelvic extractions[33]. The potential dangers of misjudging station when performing instrumental deliveries was recognized by Crichton[58] who devised an alternative method of assessing the level by estimating the proportion of the head, expressed in fifths palpable abdominally (Fig. 3.2). Engagement is defined as having occurred when not more than one-fifth of the head is palpable. Although the method is simple to perform, there are still problems with interobserver variation and a tendency to overestimate descent. Reliability of the technique may be improved by defining the clinical characteristics that are palpable at the designated levels.

5/5   The fetal head is completely palpable above the upper border of the symphysis pubis; the fingers of the examining hands can meet around the head.

4/5   The lower portion of the presenting part is just below the upper border of the symphysis pubis; the hands cannot quite meet between the fetal head and the maternal symphysis pubis.

3/5   The occipitofrontal diameter of the head may

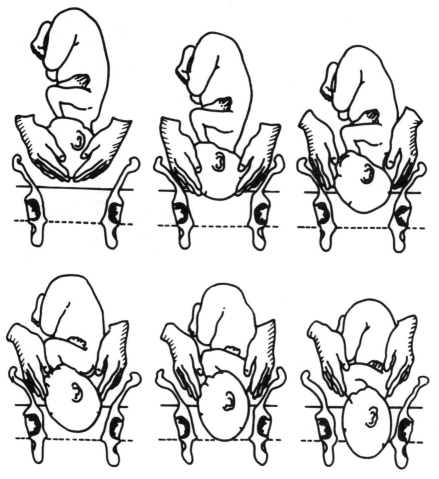

Fig. 3.2 Estimating the level of the head in 'fifths'

be palpated just above the upper border of the symphysis pubis.

2/5 The head is almost but not quite engaged. On one side, usually the side of the sinciput, the head may be easily palpable while on the other, the side of the occiput, it may not be so easily palpable.

1/5 The fetal head is just engaged; the head, usually the sinciput, may be palpated with the fingers on one side only. The occiput cannot be palpated below the upper border of the symphysis pubis.

0/5 The head is deeply engaged; neither the occiput nor the sinciput are palpable below the upper border of the symphysis pubis.

Differentiating the level of a fetal head that has not quite engaged (2/5) from one that has just engaged (1/5) may not always be easy but the distinction is important if vacuum extraction is being considered. The lower abdomen and uterus may become tender during a long labour. Palpation may cause the mother discomfort, tempting her to resist the examination. However, if she is forewarned and the examination performed gently, she may be able to assist the examiner by consciously relaxing the muscles of the abdominal wall to allow a more accurate assessment to be made. The problem of making a wrong diagnosis of engagement can be reduced by considering both the number of fifths of head palpable abdominally and the findings obtained by vaginal examination. Bimanual palpation may reveal more head palpable above the symphysis pubis than is detected by abdominal palpation alone.

Position of the head

Position of the head should be determined as accurately as possible because localization of the flexion point and correct application of the cup depend upon it. When the fetal head is in the mid pelvis, occipitoposterior and lateral positions are common and are associated with varying degrees of deflexion and asynclitism[59]. Although assessment of position is most reliable when the fontanelles and sutures are palpated by vaginal examination, it may be difficult to distinguish the anterior from the posterior fontanelle when pronounced moulding or a large caput succedaneum are present. In such circumstances, palpation of an ear may help to orientate the position of the head in the pelvis, but the manoeuvre is not always easy to perform and may cause discomfort for the mother unless appropriate analgesia has been administered. If the findings on vaginal examination are inconclusive, abdominal palpation may help to establish on which side of the mother's abdomen the fetal back is situated and so indicate the side of the occiput. Similarly, provided the head has not become deeply engaged, the sinciput may also be palpable behind one or other pubic ramus and help to locate the position of the anterior fontanelle. Because the diagnosis may be less certain at the time of the procedure for reasons mentioned above, position of the head should be established early during the course of labour whenever abdominal or vaginal examination is performed. Ideally the final assessment should be undertaken by an experienced attendant, preferably by the person who will be responsible for vacuum extraction should operative assistance become necessary.

If position is still in doubt after examination, vacuum extraction should not be attempted unless the head has descended to the level of the pelvic floor or outlet.

Moulding of the head

Moulding may be used as an indication of the extent of compression to which the fetal head has been subjected during labour[60]. A method of assessing moulding has been proposed that allows

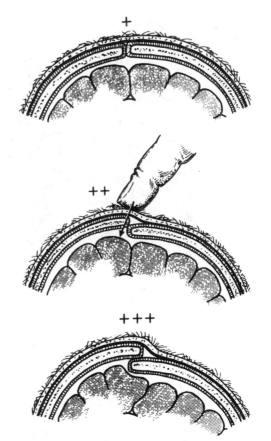

Fig. 3.3 Moulding of the head

comparison of results from one vaginal examination to another[61]. A simplication of this method is shown in Fig. 3.3. If the parietal bones are touching but not overlapping at the sagittal suture line, moulding is slight (+); if the parietal bones are overlapping but can be reduced to the normal position by finger pressure, moulding is moderate (++); and if the overlapping of the bones cannot easily be reduced, moulding is severe (+++). The degree of moulding should always be assessed before attempting operative vaginal delivery. If severe moulding is present, as is often found with deflexed and asynclitic heads in occipitoposterior and lateral positions, additional force created by applying the vacuum extractor without first correcting position and thus reducing compression of the head may increase the risk of intracranial injury[26]. Correction of the malposition and asynclitism on the other hand may often allow safe vaginal delivery but such procedures should be attempted only by experienced operators.

Recognition of cephalopelvic disproportion

Delay in the second stage of labour may be due to either cephalopelvic disproportion or inefficient uterine action. Epidural blockade associated with a reduction of maternal expulsive effort may also result in prolongation of the second stage of labour. Cephalopelvic disproportion may be defined as the inability of the fetus to pass safely through the birth canal for mechanical reasons[59]. These mechanical reasons are the relative sizes of the maternal pelvis and fetal presenting part which may vary considerably in the three dimensional size and shape and also in the degree to which the fetal head may undergo compression without injury to the brain. Disproportion may be described as either true disproportion, when even the smallest diameters of the presenting part are too big to pass through the pelvis, or relative disproportion, caused by larger presenting diameters of the head that are commonly associated with lateral and posterior positions of the occiput and which result from deflexion and asynclitism. The distinction between the two types of disproportion may be impossible to make but should be attempted because correction of the malposition in relative disproportion, either by enhancing uterine contractions or by manipulation, may allow safe vaginal delivery of the baby. Unfortunately, there is no reliable test that will diagnose cephalopelvic disproportion with certainty before the onset of labour. It may be suspected from the history of previous labours and on clinical examination or when delay occurs either in the late active phase or during the second stage of labour. Severe or increasing moulding of the head and a high presenting part that fails to descend despite strong uterine contractions are clinical findings suggestive of cephalopelvic disproportion[59]. On the other hand, relative disproportion may be diagnosed if the head has just engaged and if the occiput is posterior or lateral and the capacity of the pelvis is considered to be adequate for the size of the fetus. If steps are not taken to relieve disproportion, the labour may become obstructed and threaten the well-being of both mother and baby. Clinical signs suggesting that obstructed labour has developed include tenderness and ballooning of the lower uterine segment, formation of a retraction ring, presence of oedema of the cervix and vulva, and bloodstained urine or bleeding from the vagina.

Since the diagnosis of cephalopelvic dispropor-tion, in most cases, cannot be established unless uterine contractions are adequate, and because spontaneous rupture of the nulliparons uterus is rare, oxytocin stimulation should be tried in all nulliparae whenever there is delay in labour, provided there are no other contraindications to its use[31]. In the multipara, on the other hand, oxytocin should be used cautiously and only under close supervision because of the additional risk of rupture of the uterus. If delay in labour has advanced to the stage of obstruction, caesarean section should be the method of choice to deliver the baby. In areas where it is practised, symphysiotomy may offer an alternative in some cases of obstructed labour[62, 63].

Operator experience

To achieve good results with the vacuum extractor the operator's level of experience should be appropriately matched to the requirements of the procedure. Unfortunately, training programmes in this method of operative delivery are not common, and many users of the vacuum extractor acquire their experience through self-instruction[65, 66]. In centres where vacuum extraction is practised infrequently, lack of familiarity with the instrument may lead to inappropriate use[67, 68]. Since vacuum extractions from the outlet of the pelvis are easy to perform and safe for the fetus, inexperienced operators would be wise to master the technique at this station before attempting the more complicated mid pelvic rotational procedures or the highly challenging special uses of the instrument.

SELECTION OF PATIENTS FOR VACUUM EXTRACTION

Patients suitable for vacuum extraction may be selected on the basis of the history of the pregnancy and labour, assessment of the conditions of the fetus and mother, and evaluation of the abdominal and vaginal findings. The selection procedure should include the following steps.

Review of the history of the pregnancy and labour

 – Checking for high risk obstetric and general medical factors.

— Assessing the frequency and strength of uterine contractions and noting any contraindications to the use of oxytocin infusion.

Assessment of maternal condition

— Evaluating the physical and emotional state of the mother and her ability to participate actively in the birth.
— Reducing discomfort by administering appropriate analgesia and relieving apprehension by explanation of the results for the procedure.
— Checking the maternal blood pressure, temperature, pulse rate and fluid balance. If urine output is low, a catheter should be inserted into the bladder to determine whether the cause of the reduced output is dehydration or urethral compression by the fetal head.

Assessment of fetal well-being

— Noting the colour of the liquor for the presence of meconium or blood.
— Assessing the fetal heart rate and pattern by auscultation or continuous electronic monitoring. If fetal distress is suspected, scalp blood sampling for pH estimation may help to establish the correct diagnosis.

Abdominal examination

— Categorizing the size of the baby into small, average or large.
— Assessing the number of fifths of head palpable.
— Identifying the position of the fetal back and sinciput.
— Looking for distension of the lower uterine segment or formation of a retraction ring, indicating that labour may be obstructed.

Vaginal examination

— Estimating dilatation of the cervix and station of the presenting part.
— Grading the degree of moulding as slight, moderate or severe.
— Diagnosing position of the head and extent of deflexion and asynclitism.
— Locating the flexion point.
— Estimating the capacity of the pelvis relative to the size of the baby.

By carefully evaluating the information obtained from the examination, it is possible to select patients who are suitable for vacuum extraction and to grade the procedures according to the level of operative skill required. In practice, provided there are no other overriding factors, selection may be made by considering station of the presenting part, the degree of moulding of the head and the condition of the fetus (Table 3.2). When the fetal head is visible at the outlet of the pelvis, vacuum extraction is easily performed and the risks to the fetus are minimal. The flexion point lies within the introitus and cup application will almost always be flexing median. When the fetal head is on the pelvic floor, the procedure is also safe and should not be difficult provided the operator realizes that the flexion point may be situated to one side of the introitus and adjusts the application of the cup accordingly. Paramedian applications are a common cause of cup detachment at the outlet. For mid pelvic vacuum extractions, a higher level of operator skill is required because malposition and asynclitism are often present and the operator will need to know how to apply the cup correctly in lateral and posterior positions of the occiput. If the operator has not been trained in the technique of rotational vacuum extraction, delivery by caesarean may be the safer method. On the other hand,

Table 3.2   Selection of patients

Station	Fetal distress	Moulding	Method of delivery
Outlet	Yes or no	Slight to severe	Vacuum extraction (VE)
Pelvic floor	Yes or no	Slight to severe	Vacuum extraction (malposition occasionally)
Mid pelvis	No	Moderate	Vacuum extraction (malposition frequent)
Mid pelvis	Yes	Moderate	Trial of VE (or caesarean section)
Mid pelvis	No	Severe	Trial of VE (or caesarean section)
Mid pelvis	Yes	Severe	Caesarean section
Upper pelvis	Yes or no	Slight to severe	Caesarean section

if the operator has been trained and provided the fetus is not distressed or the degree of moulding is not more than moderate, vacuum extraction may be undertaken with confidence. If fetal distress is present, the extraction should be regarded as a trial and if some difficulty is encountered, the procedure should be abandoned promptly in favour of caesarean section. Vacuum extraction should be attempted with caution if severe moulding is present, and only if there is no other concern with fetal well-being. If, in addition, fetal distress is present, caesarean section should be the preferred method of delivery. When the head is stationed above the ischial spines, caesarean section rather than vacuum extraction should be the method chosen for delivery of the fetus[68].

4

PRELIMINARIES

CHOICE OF VACUUM CUPS

There is increasing debate among users of the vacuum extractor about the advantages and limitations of the various types of cups. The principle advantage claimed for the Bird Posterior cup over the original Malmstrom design, namely that it is more manoeuvrable and makes possible a greater number of flexing applications[9], receives support from observational data[26] but has not been tested in the context of a randomized controlled trial. Reports that the O'Neil cups can withstand greater oblique traction force than either the Malmstrom or Bird cups[8], were not substantiated in a randomized comparison of the Malmstrom and O'Neil cups involving 410 women at term with a healthy singleton fetus[69]. No differences were found between the two types of cups except that failure to deliver was more frequent in women allocated to the O'Neil cup (3 per cent) than in women allocated to the Malmstrom cup (0.5 per cent). Both instruments had a high success rate which probably relates to the fact that vacuum extraction was conducted as an elective procedure. For this reason, results should be interpreted with caution as they may not apply to all indicated deliveries[70].

The New Generation cups, Anterior and Posterior have been compared in a randomized controlled trial with the original Bird cups[71]. The study provided no evidence that using the New Generation cups had any advantages over the standard Bird cups, although the small sample size and broad measures of outcome would not be expected to give other than an imprecise estimate of possible differential effects. Operators' preferences were equally divided between the two types of cups despite the fact that more were familiar with the original designs. Some thought that the

new cord system made traction easier while others commented that it tended to get lost in the vagina or under the cup and preferred the chain traction mechanism because the handle could be moved closer to the cup as the head descended. The smooth dome of the New Generation Posterior cup effectively reduces the depth of the cup and some operators feel that this makes application easier when the space between fetal head and maternal sacrum or pelvic side wall is restricted.

Two models of the Soft cups, the Silastic and Mityvac have been compared in a randomized trial[72]. The Mityvac cup was more successful in achieving vaginal delivery and resulted in fewer scalp injuries. There was no significant difference in the incidence of cephalhaematoma in the two groups. As the number of women in the study was small, the results should be interpreted cautiously. Larger studies are needed to demonstrate differences in terms of significant neonatal morbidity and to assess which of the instruments is more likely to succeed with deflexed heads or malposition[73]. Reports from non-randomized studies involving soft vacuum extractor cups suggested that the cups were inefficient instruments when the fetal head was mid pelvic[74] or malpositioned[75, 76]. In theory, soft cups would appear to be less effective than metal cups because their larger size and bell-shaped design may make it difficult to manoeuvre the cup to the correct application site. Recent randomized controlled comparisons between soft and metal cups have confirmed that the soft cups have higher failure rates especially in malpositions of the head[77, 78, 79]. No differences were reported between the two groups in terms of maternal injury but differences were reported in the findings of minor neonatal injury. Although these differences did not reach significance, there was a trend towards more phototherapy and scalp injury but fewer low Apgar scores in babies delivered by metal cups[14]. The incidences of neonatal injury varied considerably between the studies, but the rates were unusually high in all of them. Lacerations were reported in 82 per cent of the babies delivered with the metal cup and 42 per cent of the Silastic group[77], frequencies that appear to be high even allowing for the fact that the majority of the lacerations were of a minor nature. Classification of neonatal injury may be difficult due to interobserver variation and differences in the definitions of severity of trauma[78]. Cephalhaematoma was defined as major trauma[77] but it is a common finding after birth, rarely develops complications and follows a transient course. Although most of the injuries that occur are minor and of little clinical significance, the cosmetic appearances are understandably a source of concern for the parents. Birth attendants should allay parental fears by reassuring them of the benign and transient nature of the chignon, cup marking and superficial scalp lesions.

For outlet and mid pelvic vacuum extractions and when the position of the occiput is anterior, all models of the vacuum cup are satisfactory as long as the operator is familiar with the instrument. For rotational extractions, the instrument of choice is a cup that incorporates the posterior design principle provided the operator has been trained in its use. Posterior cups, however, may be difficult to apply correctly when the occiput is anterior. Operators should understand how the specific modifications enhance the manoeuvrability of the cups and how these features may be used to achieve flexing median applications in all positions of the occiput. If cups are applied in an indiscriminate manner to the most accessible part of the head that is presenting within the introitus and are not placed over the correct site, it may be anticipated that the performances and outcomes of all cups will be similar irrespective of design. Because technique of application and traction may also vary with the model of the cup, obstetricians should limit the number of cups they use and become completely familiar with them. Despite the recommendation that the largest size of the Malmstrom or Bird cup should be used[3, 80] nearly all the vacuum extractions may be performed with the 50 mm cup[2]. A policy of selective use of a soft cup as first-line vacuum extractor for straightforward delivery and a metal cup if difficulty is anticipated or if rotation is required, has been proposed[81]. Such a policy has been tested in a randomized controlled trial and the preliminary results are encouraging (Johanson 1991, personal communication). If vacuum extraction is restricted to pelvic floor or outlet procedures, the soft cups appear to have advantages because they are easy to use and may cause less scalp marking than the rigid cups. On the other hand, since the soft cups are more likely to fail in mid pelvic occipitoposterior and lateral positions or when deflexion and asynclitism are present, it would seem reasonable not to use them in such circumstances[14]. Obstetricians at the start of their training who intend to use the vacuum extractor for rotational procedures will be well advised to develop confidence and skill in the use of the metal Anterior cups for outlet and non-rotational mid pelvic procedures because the basic technique of vacuum extraction is similar in all positions once the cup has been applied correctly to the head. The experience thus gained with the Anterior cup will prove invaluable when the more complex rotational operations are attempted using a Posterior cup.

ANALGESIA AND EPISIOTOMY

Appropriate analgesia should be offered to the mother before vacuum extraction is attempted. When vacuum extraction is performed by experienced operators, there should be little pain or discomfort from the procedure for the mother. Outlet vacuum extractions and extractions from the level of the pelvic floor require no analgesia unless episiotomy is performed. With few exceptions, perineal infiltration with local anaesthetic agents suffices for non-rotational and rotational vacuum extractions from the mid pelvis but some operators prefer to use pudendal block with these procedures. For low vacuum extractions episiotomy is required only for the usual obstetric indications but, for procedures from the mid pelvis, episiotomy should be performed when the head descends to the pelvic floor in order to make it easier for the operator to direct traction more posteriorly in line with the axis of the pelvis. Epidural analgesia should not be implemented for the purpose of vacuum extraction because it is not necessary and because it may reduce maternal expulsive effort. However, if the mother has already received epidural analgesia for pain relief during the course of the labour and vacuum extraction is undertaken, the operator should help her to compensate for the loss of the sensation to push by telling her when she is bearing down effectively and offering encouragement throughout the procedure. Injury to the fetus is more likely to occur if the operator substitutes increased traction for decreased maternal expulsive effort. General anaesthesia should not be employed with vacuum extraction because the strength of the uterine contractions are diminished and maternal expulsive effort is abolished.

POSITION OF THE MOTHER

Although maternal posture during the second stage of labour has been shown to have little effect on the incidence of operative delivery or perineal trauma[43], there does appear to be some benefit for the fetus if the supine position is avoided for long periods in labour[82]. Even a lateral tilt of 15 degrees was shown to improve the fetal acid-base status when compared with the supine position[83]. The lithotomy position with a wedge under one maternal buttock to produce some lateral tilt is recommended for vacuum extraction. In this position, location of the flexion point and correct application of the cup is most readily achieved. Some operators prefer the left lateral position[84] but this should be used only when the station of the head is low. Similarly the dorsal position is suitable only if the head is visible on the perineum because the direction of pull is restricted unless the buttocks can be elevated or the end of the bed lowered. When the mother has been assisted into the lithotomy position, the buttocks should extend as far as or slightly beyond the end of the bed to allow traction to be directed downward towards the floor if necessary (Fig. 4.1). The leg supports should be angled so that the thighs are comfortably flexed when the mother's buttocks overlap the end of the bed. She should be instructed in the method of pushing in this position and reinforcing the bearing down effort by grasping either the back of her thighs or, if possible, the metal poles supporting her legs. With appropriate explanation and encouragement, mothers quickly adapt to pushing in this position. Sustained bearing down is the preferred method for vacuum extraction rather than the shorter more frequent efforts. During the expulsion stage, the mother's head should be supported comfortably on pillows or by the hand of the support person.

COMMUNICATION BETWEEN THE MOTHER AND OPERATOR

During labour

If the obstetrician has not been involved in the patient's antenatal care, he or she should attempt to meet all women and their partners early in labour as an introductory visit and then at regular intervals during the course of their labour. It is not satisfactory for a woman to meet the operator for the first time when instrumental delivery is required. The mother should be kept fully informed by the birth attendant about progress of the labour and the condition of her baby and be provided with explanations for any interventions or treatments that may be prescribed. Development of a rapport between mother and obstetrician will be helpful if, later in the labour, vacuum extraction becomes necessary.

Before the procedure

If a decision is made to expedite the birth of the baby and circumstances are suitable for vacuum

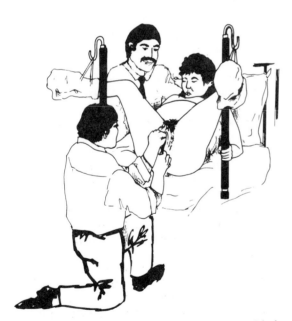

Fig. 4.1 The mother in the lithotomy position with the buttocks reaching to the end of the bed. The operator is using the finger-thumb technique and by kneeling is able to direct traction downwards

extraction, the obstetrician should spend a short time explaining to the parents the reasons for the decision and the options available for subsequent management. A brief description of vacuum extraction in non-technical terms should be offered to the couple using a fetal mannequin to explain such findings as malposition or deflexion and to demonstrate the basic principles. It should be emphasized to the mother that birth will result largely from her own expulsive powers and that the operator's role with the vacuum extractor will be complementary to her efforts. She should be informed that the duration of the procedure will last not longer than 15 minutes and that, if any difficulty is encountered, delivery will be completed by caesarean section in the interests of the baby. Such simple explanations will help to relieve the couple's anxiety and gain the mother's confidence and cooperation.

During the procedure

While preparations are being made for cleansing and draping the perineum and for providing adequate pain relief, the mother should be encouraged to practise pushing while in the lithotomy position during each contraction. The obstetrician should communicate frequently with the mother, advising her when she is pushing correctly and urging her to produce maximum expulsive effort. If epidural analgesia has been administered, the operator should help to compensate for the absence of the desire to bear down by telling the mother when the expulsive efforts are effective and informing her of the progress that she is making.

At some stage during the interval between contractions, the operator should mention that when the cup is removed from the baby's head after the birth is completed, there will be a harmless swelling of the scalp that will decrease in size over one or two hours leaving a circular mark which may take a few days to disappear completely. The extent to which parents will be reassured and accept the appearance of a baby after vacuum extraction will be influenced by the attitude and explanations of the operator and birth attendants.[65]

POSITION OF THE OPERATOR

After the cup has been correctly applied to the fetal head, and while awaiting the onset of a uterine contraction before the start of traction, the operator should be seated on a stool and remain seated until the head has descended to the level of the pelvic outlet. The sitting position will encourage the operator to exert traction in a downward direction and assist descent of the presenting part by maintaining the flexion point on or just behind the axis of the pelvis (see *Traction*, p. 23). For low extractions or when the head has descended to the outlet, the direction of traction will change progressively upwards until the standing position becomes more appropriate. For rotational extractions from the mid pelvis, the operator may find it easier to direct traction towards the floor by getting down on one knee for the initial pull (see Fig. 4.1, on p. 40). Eye to eye contact should be maintained between mother and operator at all times so that communication and interaction may occur freely.

5

PROCEDURE

STANDARD PROCEDURE FOR VACUUM EXTRACTION

When a valid indication for vacuum extraction exists, the procedure should include the following steps.

Review of pregnancy and labour

A check of the history for high risk factors should be made and the condition of the fetus, the state of the mother and her ability to push effectively and the strength of the uterine contractions should be assessed. Syntocinon infusion should be commenced if there is suspicion of hypototic uterine action provided there are no contraindications to its use.

Abdominal examination

The level of the head should be carefully assessed and the position of the fetal back and sinciput identified.

Vaginal examination

Dilatation of the cervix, station of the presenting part and the degree of moulding are assessed. The position of the head should be established and the extent of deflexion and asynclitism noted.

Selection of patients suitable for vacuum extraction

By evaluating the findings from the history and examination it is possible to select candidates suitable for vacuum extraction and to grade the procedures into lower and higher risk groups (see Table 3.2).

Informing the mother

The operator should start by explaining briefly to the mother the reasons for the procedure and discuss with her the alternative methods of management. If a decision is made to proceed with vacuum extraction, the mother should understand that her participation is an integral part of the procedure and that delivery will occur largely as a result of her expulsive effort rather than vacuum extraction. She should also be advised that the procedure will not last longer than 15 minutes.

Testing the vacuum system

The operator or an assistant should check the pump to ensure that there are no leakages in the system.

Position of the mother

The mother should be assisted into the lithotomy position and a wedge placed under one buttock to produce some lateral tilt. The buttocks should extend slightly beyond the end of the bed to allow traction to be directed downwards towards the floor. She should be encouraged to practice pushing in this position during the preparations for vacuum extraction.

Preparation of the vulva

The vulva is prepared and draped in the usual manner. A catheter need be passed only if the woman is unable to void or if the bladder is visibly or palpably distended.

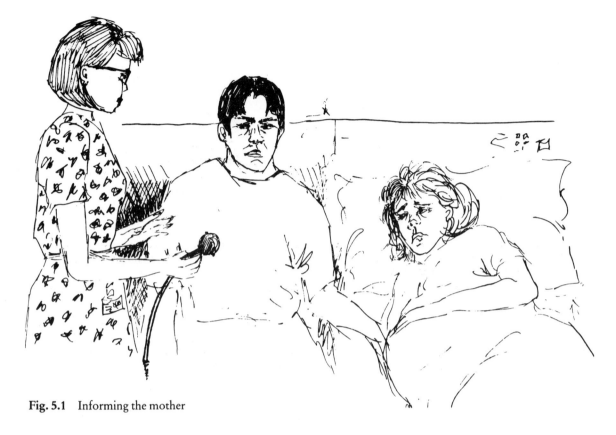

Fig. 5.1 Informing the mother

Analgesia

Perineal infiltration with a local anaesthetic agent will suffice for the majority of vacuum extractions, but some operators prefer to use pudendal block. If epidural analgesia has been administered, it is important that the mother be instructed in the technique of bearing down effectively with each contraction.

METHOD OF LOCALIZING THE FLEXION POINT

Before applying the cup to the fetal head, the position of the occiput is rechecked and the flexion point is located. To localize the position of the flexion point, two observations are required: the estimated distance from the flexion point to the posterior fourchette; and the degree of lateral displacement of the flexion point from the midline axis of the pelvis. These observations should be made during the vaginal examination conducted as part of the assessment of labour.

To estimate the distance of the flexion point from the posterior fourchette

If the tip of the examining finger is placed on the flexion point, the distance to the posterior fourchette may be calculated by measuring the length of the finger from the tip to where it makes contact with the fourchette. This estimate may be made with sufficient accuracy for practical purposes if it is known that the distance from the tip of the middle finger to the proximal interphalangeal joint is 5 to 6 cms (Fig. 5.2) and to the metacarpophalangeal joint, 10 to 11 cms (Fig. 5.3). By observing the finger-length from the fourchette to the flexion point, the operator can estimate how far the centre of the cup must be inserted into the birth canal to achieve a flexing application. The distance will vary with station, position and degree of asynclit-

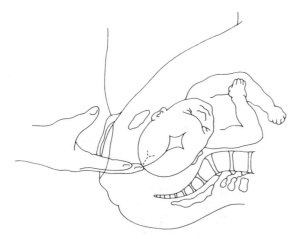

Fig. 5.2   Estimating the distance from the flexion point to the posterior fourchette in low-mid pelvic stations. The distance from the tip of the finger to the proximal interphalangeal joint is 5–6 cms

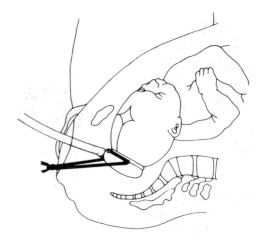

Fig. 5.4   Estimating the cup insertion distance by observing the length of cord or chain protruding from the vagina

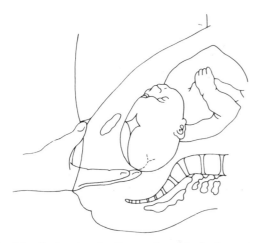

Fig. 5.3   Estimating the distance from the flexion point to the posterior fourchette in mid pelvic stations. The distance from the tip of the finger to the metacarpophalangeal joint is 10–11 cms

ism of the head but in the mid pelvic occipitoposterior and occipitolateral positions, the flexion point may be a complete finger's length (10 to 11 cms) from the posterior fourchette. Operators will find this information helpful when using a Posterior cup because these estimated finger distances can be extrapolated into cord or chain lengths and give an accurate indication of how far to insert the cup. For instance, if the total length of cord from the centre of the cup to the knot is

known (see Fig. 1.22b, p. 9), the length of cord visible outside the vulva will indicate to the operator if the cup has been inserted the correct distance (Fig. 5.4).

To determine the distance of the flexion point from the midline axis

The location of the flexion point in relation to the midline axis may be determined by a two-handed technique. The tip of the index finger of the left hand is placed under the symphysis pubis and marks the midline reference position while the right hand identifies the flexion point as previously described (Fig. 5.5). By observing the distance between finger tips, the operator is able to visualize the extent of lateral displacement or rotation of the flexion point.

When the fetal head is stationed at the outlet or on the pelvic floor and the sagittal suture lies in the anteroposterior plane, the flexion point will be located in the midline and situated on the part of the head that is presenting within the introitus. In these circumstances, direct application of a vacuum cup will achieve a flexing median application. In obliquely anterior positions of the head, the flexion point is usually palpable within the introitus but will be observed to be lateral rather than anterior when related to the midpoint of the pubic arch (Fig. 5.6). In these positions, unless the cup is manoeuvred to take into account the displacement

ESTIMATING THE DISPLACEMENT OF THE FLEXION POINT FROM THE MIDLINE

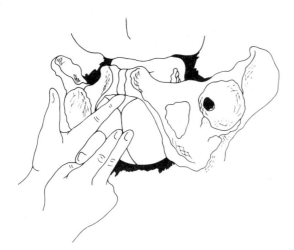

Fig 5.5   In direct occipitoanterior positions

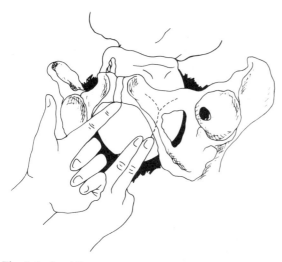

Fig. 5.6   In oblique occipitoanterior and occipitolateral positions

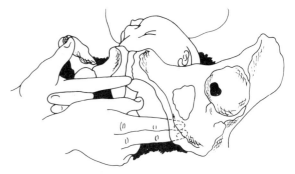

Fig. 5.7   In occipitoposterior positions

of the flexion point, application may frequently be paramedian even if the cup has been inserted far enough into the birth canal to achieve flexion. With lateral positions of the occiput, the parietal aspect of the fetal head is commonly the presenting part. It will be apparent, using the two-handed technique, that the flexion point in these positions will often be situated behind the caput succedaneum which forms mainly over the parietal bone. If the fetal head is well flexed, the location of

the flexion point will be near the midline and correct application of the cup will be achieved as long as the cup is inserted far enough into the mother's pelvis. If, on the other hand, the fetal head is not well flexed, the flexion point will be closer to the sidewall of the pelvis and the application will be deflexing and paramedian unless appropriate correction is made.

Displacement of the flexion point from the midline is most pronounced when the occiput is obliquely posterior (Fig. 5.7). In this position, some degree of deflexion and asynclitism of the fetal head is often present. If the vacuum extractor is used for rotational procedures, the operator should know how to locate the exact position of the flexion point using the two-handed technique and be able to manoeuvre the centre of the cup until it is over the flexion point. Failure to do so will result in deflexing and/or paramedian applications in a number of cases. With practice, the time to identify the flexion point, estimate the distance from the posterior fourchette and assess the degree of lateral displacement should take only a matter of seconds. When the examination is completed, however, there should be no doubt in the operator's mind of the exact location of the flexion point and the ideal application site of the cup.

Application of the cup

Choice of vacuum cup

The Malmstrom and Anterior cups and all the Soft cups are suitable if the occiput is anterior but a

Posterior cup should be used for lateral and posterior positions of the occiput.

Applying the cup

An assistant connects the distal end of the cup tubing to the length of tubing from the vacuum pump. The operator smears the outside of the cup lightly with obstetric cream and, having forewarned the mother, retracts the perineum with two fingers to form a space into which the cup is inserted gently in one movement. The cup is pressed against the fetal head and manoeuvred until its centre lies over the flexion point. In anterior positions, while one hand holds the cup in position, the index finger of the other hand is swept around the rim of the cup to check that there is no maternal tissue or fetal electrode trapped between cup and scalp. Because it is usually impossible to reach behind a correctly placed cup in occipitolateral and posterior positions, some operators omit this check.

Inducing the vacuum

When the operator is satisfied that the application is correct, a vacuum pressure of 0.2 kgms/cm^2 is induced and the cup position rechecked before increasing the vacuum in one step to the recommended pressure of 0.8 kgms/cm^2. The cup is correctly positioned when a distance of 3 cms or more can be palpated between the anterior fontanelle and the leading edge of the cup and the sagittal suture may be felt to pass under the middle of the cup. Traction should be delayed for two minutes to allow the chignon to form although gentle traction may be commenced sooner if necessary.

Method of traction

Attachment of the cup to the scalp is most effective when the direction of pull is perpendicular to the cup[3]. This is nearly always possible for low extractions but, for mid pelvic rotational procedures, oblique traction is often necessary to keep the axis of the fetal head in line with the pelvic axis. Oblique traction, however, predisposes to cup detachment which may cause injury to the scalp. To counteract this tendency, traction should be a two-handed exercise with the right hand holding the traction handle and pulling in the direction of descent (Fig. 5.8). The thumb of the non-pulling hand presses against the dome of the cup and helps to prevent complete detachment from the scalp while the index finger of the same hand rests on the scalp in front of the cup and monitors descent of the head. This finger-thumb position of the non-pulling hand should be maintained as long as traction is applied especially if the direction of pull is oblique, or until the head is crowned. It has been suggested that the left hand in the finger-thumb position should exert backward pressure on the fetal head towards the sacrum to promote axis traction at the same time as pulling during a contraction[24] and that descent may be enhanced by a series of pendulum or rocking movements from side to side[85]. Such manoeuvres should be exercised with caution because the oblique directional force may increase the predisposition to cup detachment especially if application is incorrect or if force is excessive. Traction is applied at the onset of a contraction and is maintained smoothly for the duration thereof. The operator should offer constant encouragement to the mother to bear down and should inform her of the progress being made. During the procedure the fetal heart should be monitored regularly by an assistant. The first pull should cause flexion of the head and some descent. By the end of the second pull the head should be on the pelvic floor and with the third pull delivery of the head should be complete or

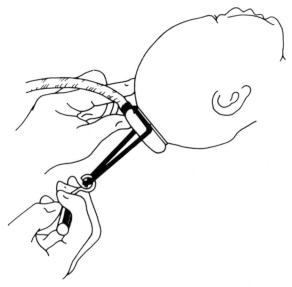

Fig. 5.8   Method of traction: finger-thumb position

imminent. If epidural analgesia has been administered, however, one or two gentle pulls may help the mother to become accustomed to pushing effectively in the absence of bearing-down sensations. Traction is discontinued between contractions or if an audible hiss is heard signalling loss of vacuum. After delivery of the head, the vacuum is released, the cup eased off the scalp and the birth completed in the normal manner.

Procedures using the Soft cups, the Anterior and Posterior cups are described in separate sections. These descriptions and illustrations apply to right-handed operators.

After the delivery

The operator should examine the baby immediately after the birth for scalp injury and to note cup application site. This information should be recorded with other details of the procedure on a suitable data form (Table 5.1). If difficulty was encountered during the extraction, regular inspections of the scalp should be made to exclude bleeding into the subgaleal space. At delivery, the parents should be informed and reassured that the chignon will disappear in a matter of hours and that marking from the cup will leave no traces after a few days. On the day after delivery, the operator should re-examine the baby in the mother's presence to allay any concerns and to discuss the reasons for the procedure.

TECHNIQUE USING SOFT CUPS

The Silastic cup	(Figs 5.9–5.14)
The Silc cup	(Figs 5.15–5.19)
The Mityvac and CMI cups	(Figs 5.20–5.24)

Application of the cup

The soft cups are grasped near the broad end and compressed between the thumb and fingers of the right hand to make insertion through the introitus easier (Fig. 5.9). The index and middle fingers of the other hand should be inserted into the introitus to retract the perineum (Fig. 5.10) and create a space into which the cup is inserted with a single, gentle movement immediately following a contraction. The cup is then manoeuvred laterally until its centre lies over the flexion point or until the elastic resistance of the vulval tissues prevents further movement (Fig. 5.11). Because the fetal head is

Table 5.1 Vacuum extraction data form

SELECTION DATA
- Indication for vacuum extraction – fetal distress, failure to progress, elective shortening of the second stage
- Maternal analgesia
- Strength of uterine contractions
- Use of oxytocin infusion
- Maternal ability to bear down
- Station of the fetal head
- Dilatation of the cervix
- Degree of moulding
- Extent of caput formation
- Position of the fetal head

PROCEDURAL DATA
- Type and size of vacuum cup
- Number of pulls to complete delivery
- Did the cup become detached? If so, number of times?
- Type of cup application achieved – flexing median, flexing paramedian, deflexing median or deflexing paramedian
- Rotation of the head (in malpositions) – autorotation, manual rotation, forceps rotation, failure of rotation
- Did the allocated cup complete the delivery?
- Was there a change to another instrument – forceps or vacuum?
- Was caesarean section required to complete the delivery?
- Reasons why the vacuum extractor did not complete the delivery – inability to apply cup, no descent of the head, detachment of the cup, equipment fault
- Operator status – obstetrician, senior registrar, registrar, resident, midwife

OUTCOME DATA – MATERNAL
- Episiotomy
- Injury to perineum, vagina, cervix
- Injury to sphincter, anus, rectum

OUTCOME DATA – NEONATAL
- Condition of the infant at birth
- Scalp effects – chignon, marking, bruising, blistering, abrasion, cephalhaematoma, subcutaneous haematoma, subgaleal haematoma
- Neonatal course – jaundice, phototherapy, neurological state, retinal haemorrhage, condition of infant on discharge from hospital

usually completely flexed when it is at the level of the outlet or on the pelvic floor, the cup will nearly always cover the posterior fontanelle. The finger is then gently passed around the rim of the cup to ensure that no maternal tissue has been inadver-

THE SOFT CUPS

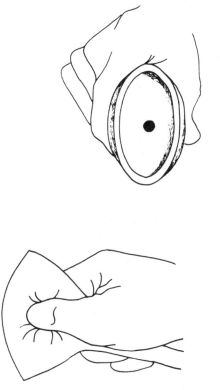

Fig. 5.9 Compressing the cup to make insertion easier

tently drawn beneath the edges of the cup and to check that the cup has been correctly applied to the fetal head.

Inducing the vacuum

With the cup pressed against the fetal head, a partial vacuum of 0.2 kgms/cm^2 is induced and the operator should once again palpate around the edges of the cup with one finger to recheck that no maternal tissues have been trapped under the cup and to confirm that cup application is correct. The partial vacuum may then be increased in one step to the recommended working pressure of 0.8 kgms/cm^2. Traction with the Soft cups may be commenced at the onset of the next contraction as soon as the desired vacuum pressures have been achieved. With the CMI vacuum pump, the negative pressure may be reduced between contractions and increased again at the commencement of the next contraction.

Traction

Traction should be synchronized with uterine contractions. It should be applied with two hands, one gripping the handle and pulling, while the other hand rests against the fetal head and edge of the cup in order to check that the head and not just the scalp is descending when traction is applied. If descent of the fetal head does not occur with traction, the operator should check that the direction of traction is correct. Traction should be exerted parallel to the birth canal with the handle of the cup as straight as possible and should be applied smoothly through the contraction (Fig. 5.12). An audible hiss is heard if the adhesive force is about to be exceeded as air is sucked under the cup during traction. Further traction will result in complete separation of the cup from the fetal head. If this occurs, traction should be discontinued and the cup allowed to adhere firmly again. The direction of pull may require adjustment before traction is resumed during the next contraction. In obliquely anterior positions of the occiput, rotation to the direct anterior position will be completed as the head descends to the level of the outlet of the pelvis (Fig. 5.13). When the cup is used for rotation, the marker lines or ridges on some of the cups serve as directional guides. As the head begins to crown, traction is changed to an upward direction at an angle of 45 degrees to the floor (Fig. 5.14). Episiotomy may be performed as indicated. When the head is delivered, traction is ceased, the suction is released and delivery completed in the usual manner.

THE SILASTIC CUP

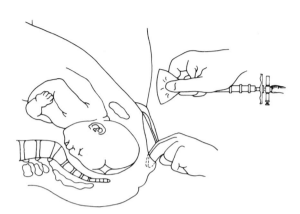

Fig. 5.10 Retracting the perineum and inserting the cup

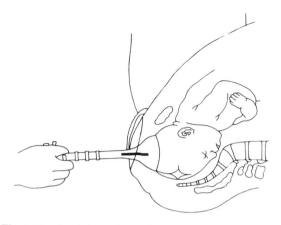

Fig. 5.12 Applying axis traction

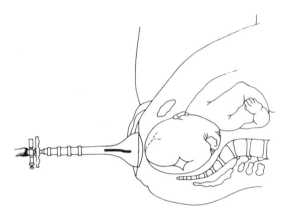

Fig. 5.11 Placing the cup over the flexion point

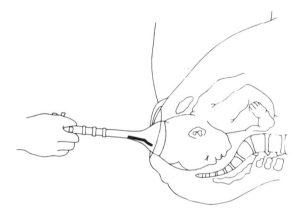

Fig. 5.13 Changing the direction of traction

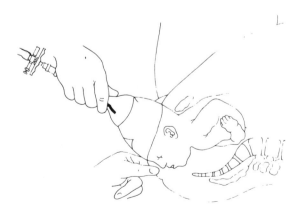

Fig. 5.14 Delivering the head

THE SILC CUP

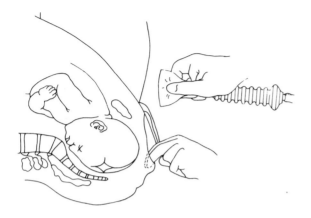

Fig. 5.15   Retracting the perineum and inserting the cup

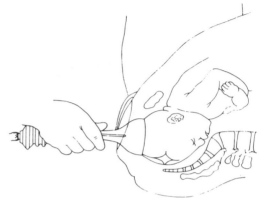

Fig. 5.17   Applying axis traction

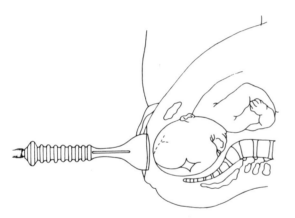

Fig. 5.16   Placing the cup over the flexion point

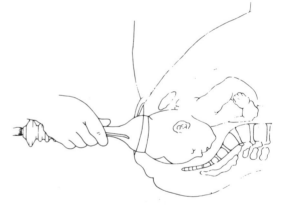

Fig. 5.18   Changing the direction of traction

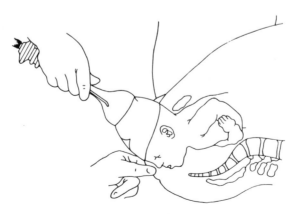

Fig. 5.19   Delivering the head

THE CMI (SOFT TOUCH) CUP

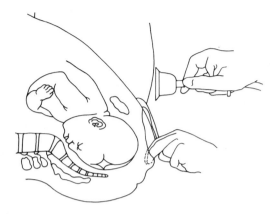

Fig. 5.20 Retracting the perineum and inserting the cup

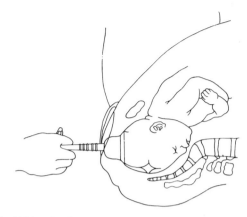

Fig. 5.22 Applying axis traction

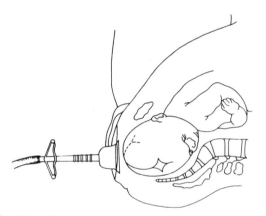

Fig. 5.21 Placing the cup over the flexion point

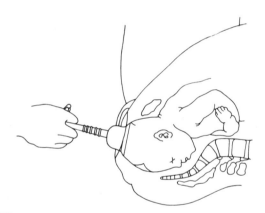

Fig. 5.23 Changing the direction of traction

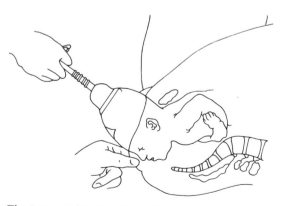

Fig. 5.24 Delivering the head

TECHNIQUE USING ANTERIOR CUPS

The Malmstrom cup   (Figs 5.25–5.29)
The Bird and O'Neil cups   (Figs 5.30–5.35)

Application of the cup

The Malmstrom and Anterior cups (Bird and O'Neil) are held in the right hand with the thumb and forefinger grasping the suction nozzle near where it joins the dome of the cup (Fig. 5.25). The tubing and traction chain or cord of the Anterior cups are also held between the fingers and palm of the hand (see Fig. 5.30). The Anterior cup, with its eccentric tubal attachment, should be orientated in such a way that the centre of the cup is below the level of the tube. The labia are separated and the perineum retracted to facilitate insertion of the cup. The outside of the cup is lightly smeared with obstetric cream and gently inserted by turning it slightly sideways and tilted backwards so that the smooth, rounded edge of the lower part of the cup presses against the perineal tissues. Once insertion is completed, the cup should sit comfortably in the space between the fetal head and maternal perineum (Fig. 5.26). The cup is pressed lightly against the fetal head and moved in the direction of the flexion point until it is positioned correctly or until the tubing prevents further lateral movement. The eccentric attachment of the tubing of the anterior cup design allows the centre of the cup to be rotated closer to the flexion point, using the tube as the pivot. While one hand holds the cup in the desired position, the index finger of the other hand is swept around the margin of the cup to ensure that no maternal tissue has been trapped beneath the cup.

Inducing the vacuum

When the operator is satisfied that the cup has been applied correctly to the scalp, a vacuum pressure of 0.2 kgms/cm^2 should be induced. This will cause light attachment of the cup to the scalp while a finger may be passed around it to re-check that neither cervical nor vaginal tissue is interposed between the cup and the scalp. This exercise should be performed with care in order not to displace the cup. When the operator has confirmed that the application is flexing median, the vacuum pressure may be increased to the recommended pressure of 0.8 kgms/cm^2 in one step. At this stage, it is advisable to wait for two minutes to allow a chignon to form before applying traction to the cup.

Traction

Traction should involve both hands, with the thumb of the non-pulling hand pressing firmly against the dome of the cup and keeping the operator in touch with the cup while helping to prevent it from slipping off the scalp. The index finger of the same hand, resting on the scalp in front of the cup, monitors descent (Fig. 5.27). While traction is applied smoothly throughout a contraction, the mother is encouraged to push for the duration unless this is contraindicated. Traction should be discontinued between contractions or if loss of vacuum occurs. Oblique traction, by tending to depress one side of the cup and raising the opposite one, may lever the cup from its attachment to the scalp. Traction should therefore be perpendicular to the cup's surface but this may not always be possible if the cup is used in malpositions of the head. Traction should be directed more anteriorly as the head advances down the birth canal, but as far as possible should remain perpendicular to the cup (Fig. 5.28). As the head begins to crown, traction is directed upwards to assist delivery by extension (Fig. 5.29). Once the head is born, the cup should be detached by releasing the vacuum following which birth is completed in the usual manner.

THE MALMSTROM CUP

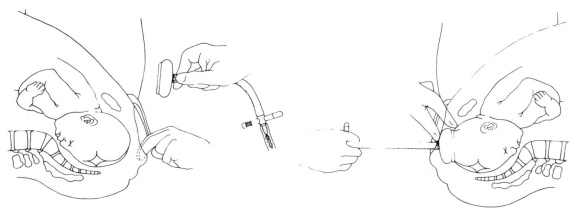

Fig. 5.25 Retracting the perineum and inserting the cup

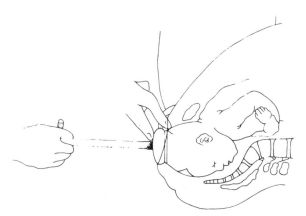

Fig. 5.27 Applying axis traction

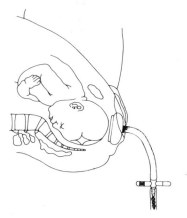

Fig. 5.26 Placing the cup over the flexion point

Fig. 5.28 Changing the direction of traction

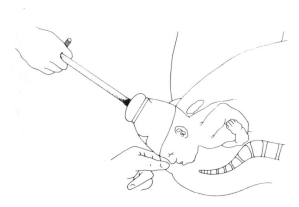

Fig. 5.29 Delivering the head

THE ANTERIOR CUP

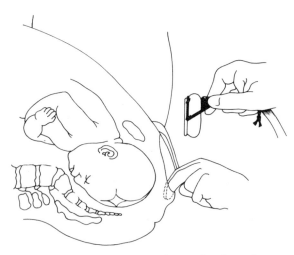

Fig. 5.30 Holding the cup and retracting the perineum

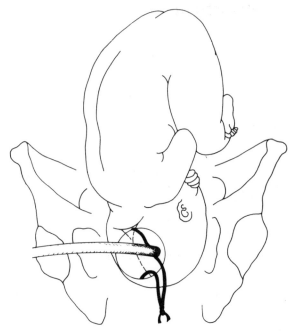

Fig. 5.32(a) Correct application

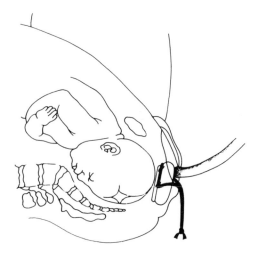

Fig. 5.31 Placing the cup over the flexion point

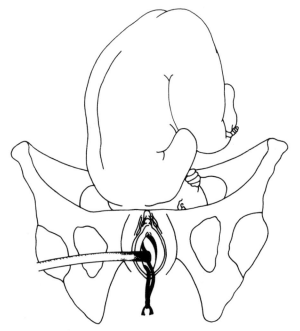

Fig. 5.32(b) The operator's view

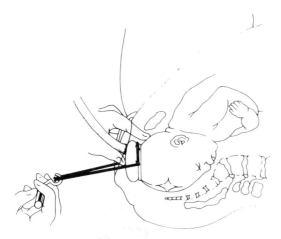

Fig. 5.33 Applying axis traction while maintaining finger-thumb position

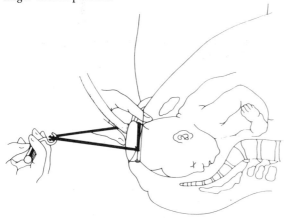

Fig. 5.34 Changing direction of traction as fetal head descends

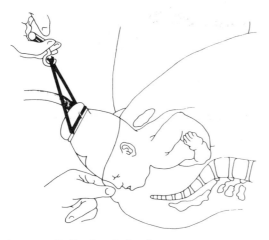

Fig. 5.35 Delivering the head

TECHNIQUE USING POSTERIOR CUPS

The Bird and O'Neil Posterior cups:

- *Occipitoposterior position* (Figs 5.36–5.47)
- *Occipitolateral position* (Figs 5.48–5.70)

Use of the Bird and O'Neil Posterior cups for occipitoposterior and lateral positions should follow the general steps outlined in the standard procedure for vacuum extraction (see p. 52). There are, however, some important differences in the techniques of applying the cup and administering traction. Although the illustrations depict the New Generation Bird cup, the technique is similar with the O'Neil cup.

Applying the Posterior cup

The Posterior cup should be held in the right hand with the thumb and index finger gripping the suction nozzle and with the tubing and suction chain or cord held in the palm of the hand (Fig. 5.36). The operator must ensure that the looped traction cord of the New Generation Bird cup does not pass under the tubing when the cup is applied, or effective traction will not be possible. The perineum is retracted by the index and middle fingers of the left hand and the cup is inserted in a single but gentle movement. Once inserted, the cup should sit comfortably in the space formed between the perineum and fetal head (Fig. 5.37). At this stage, the mother should be informed that some manoeuvring will be required to position the cup correctly over the baby's head and that, although she will be aware of the manipulations, she should not feel pain. The presence of a large caput succedaneum on the parietal aspect of the head may impede further movement of the cup towards the sacrum. To overcome this, the operator should position the left hand as shown in Fig. 5.38, touching the caput with the middle and index fingers. The pliable nature of the caput makes it possible for the fingers to lift it sufficiently to allow the advancing edge of the cup to pass under the caput. The index finger of the right hand pushes the cup as far as possible into the curve of the sacrum or until the centre of the cup is judged to be over the flexion point. In obliquely posterior positions of the occiput, it is very unusual for the cup to be inserted too far into the birth canal so the operator should strive for maximum distance. The

THE POSTERIOR CUP: USE IN OCCIPITOPOSTERIOR POSITIONS

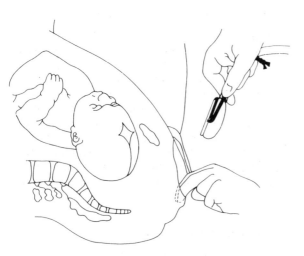

Fig. 5.36   Retracting the perineum and inserting the cup

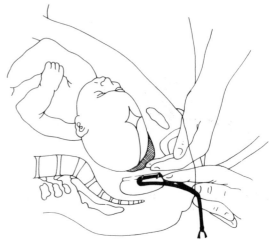

Fig. 5.38   Lifting the caput and manoeuvring the cup over the flexion point

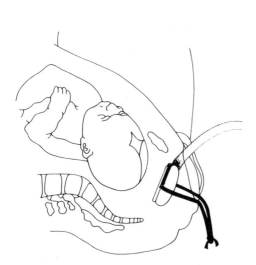

Fig. 5.37   Insertion into perineal space is completed in one movement

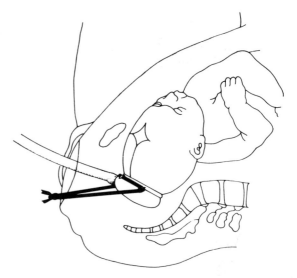

Fig. 5.39   Checking that the application is correct

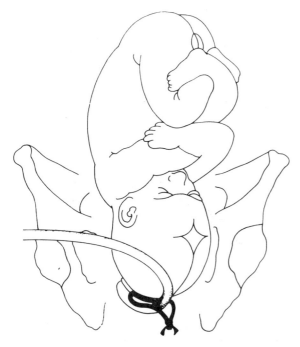

Fig. 5.40(a) Correct application

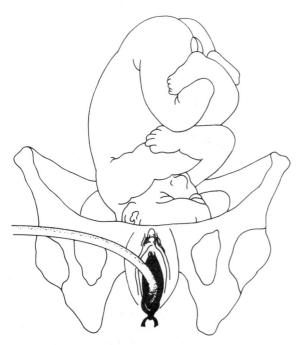

Fig. 5.40(b) The operator's view

same rule applies for some lateral positions of the occiput associated with asynclitism where the flexion point is displaced towards the sacrum. In other cases where the head descends beyond the level of the ischial spines insertion will depend on the measured distance from the flexion point to the posterior fourchette. If the flexion point is situated to one side of the midline, the cup should then be directed towards that side, taking care it does not slide outwards during the manoeuvre. When the operator is satisfied that the cup is positioned correctly, a check of the application should be made by identifying the anterior fontanelle with the index finger of the left hand, estimating that the distance along the sagittal suture to the nearest part of the cup is at least 3 cms and checking that the suture line passes inder the middle of the cup (Fig. 5.39). If the cup has been correctly applied to the head (Fig. 5.40a), in mid pelvic obliquely posterior positions of the occiput, the cup should not be visible within the introitus. The operator should see the suction tube passing over the perineum into the vagina and little more than the knot of the cord externally (Fig. 5.40b). At lower stations of the head, correspondingly more of the traction cord or chain will be visible outside the introitus. With practice, the procedure of applying the Posterior cup and inducing the vacuum should be accomplished easily in the interval between two contractions to be ready to commence gentle traction at the onset of the next contraction.

Inducing the vacuum

Once correct application has been confirmed, the index finger of the right hand should continue to hold the cup in the correct position while the vacuum is being induced (Fig. 5.41). This counteracts the tendency for the cup to be expelled by elastic resistance of the maternal tissues before the chignon can form to allow effective attachment to the scalp. Initially, a vacuum pressure of 0.2 kgm/cm^2 should be induced while the cup position is rechecked to ensure that the application is flexing median before increasing the vacuum to the recommended pressure of 0.8 kgm/cm^2. When operators develop the skill to achieve flexing median applications consistently, this intermediate step may be discarded.

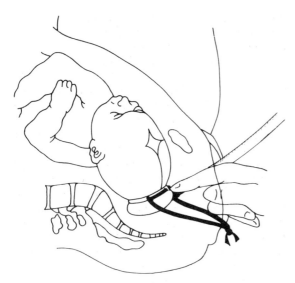

Fig. 5.41   Holding the cup in position while inducing the vacuum

Traction

The ideal (perpendicular) direction of pull is frequently not possible initially when the cup has been applied correctly to a malpositioned head stationed in the mid pelvis. This is because the presence of the perineum causes traction to be directed obliquely to the cup and increases the risk of detachment. The finger-thumb position of the left hand that has been recommended to prevent this complication is often not possible in occipito-posterior positions on the initial pull. In these circumstances, the thumb may be inserted into the vagina and pressed against the dome of the cup to offer counterpressure when traction is oblique (Fig. 5.42). Weak traction directed towards the floor will flex the head sufficiently to alter the relative position of the cup in the vagina from horizontal to vertical and allow the finger-thumb position to be adopted (Fig. 5.43). The relative shift in the position of the cup allows the operator to know that flexion has occurred by the cup becoming visible within the vagina and by the lengthening of the traction cord or chain outside the introitus. To prevent kinking at the junction with the cup, the suction tube should be supported by the operator's left hand or with the aid of an assistant.

Rotation occurs automatically as the head descends, provided the application of the cup is

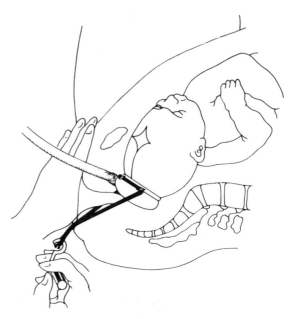

Fig. 5.42   Thumb counterpressure with initial pull while directing traction towards the floor

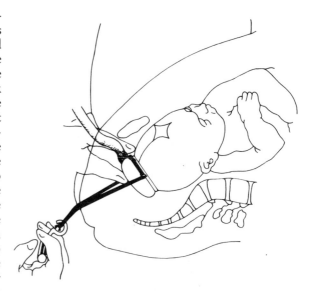

Fig. 5.43   Flexion of the head causes lengthening of the cord and enables the finger-thumb position to be adopted

correct and traction is directed in line with the axis of the pelvis. The operator may observe that autorotation is occurring by noting the change in position of the tubing where it joins the cup (Fig.

5.44). As the head rotates, the tubing will be seen to rotate with it. Because 'rotation' of the head is a three-dimensional event involving changes in flexion and synclitism as well as rotation, the extent of the revolution of the cup may appear less than one might expect.

No attempt should be made to rotate the head either digitally or by rotating the cup. Such manoeuvres are unnecessary and may dislodge the cup or cause the cup to rotate but not the head. As the cup becomes visible at the introitus, the operator should direct traction horizontally and resist the tendency to pull in an upward direction too soon (Fig. 5.45). It should be appreciated that the midpoint of the head is situated at the level of the

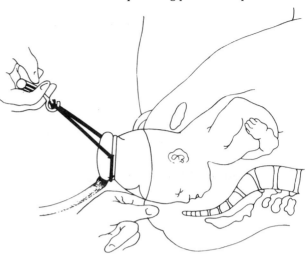

Fig. 5.46 Delivering the head

biparietal plane which is approximately 6 cms behind the cup and that the direction of pull should aim to achieve axis traction at this level. But as the head emerges from the introitus and rotation is complete, the direction of traction may be changed progressively upwards until the head has crowned and delivery is accomplished by extension (Fig. 5.46). At this point the vacuum may be released, the cup removed and delivery completed in the usual manner.

Occasionally in occipitoposterior positions of the head where extensive moulding and a large caput succedaneum are present, descent to the level of the pelvic floor may occur without autorotation. Although with further traction delivery may be accomplished in the face-to-pubis position, there may be advantages for the mother and baby for the head to be born with the occiput anterior[86]. In these circumstances, anterior rotation may still be possible at this low level using the following technique. The operator presses the thumb of the left hand against the centre of the dome of the cup to prevent too rapid descent of the head (Fig. 5.47a). The mother is then encouraged to bear down during a contraction and this expulsive force is converted into a rotary force by the thumb preventing descent while weak traction is applied in a slightly downward direction (Fig. 5.47b). With the thumb acting as the pivot point, the fetal head will often rotate to the occipitoanterior position (Fig. 5.47c). After anterior rotation, traction is directed upwards and delivery completed normally.

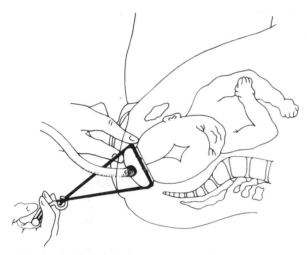

Fig. 5.44 With descent autorotation occurs

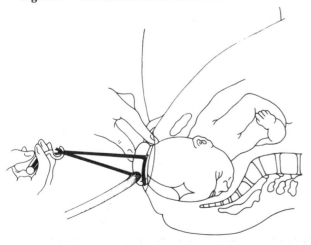

Fig. 5.45 Changing the direction of traction

ANTERIOR ROTATION AT THE OUTLET

THE POSTERIOR CUP: USE IN OCCIPITOLATERAL POSITIONS

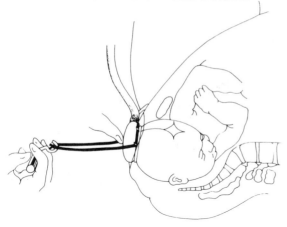

Fig. 5.47(a)   Counterpressure with the thumb

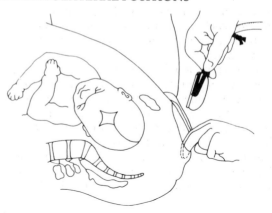

Fig. 5.48   Retracting the perineum and inserting the cup

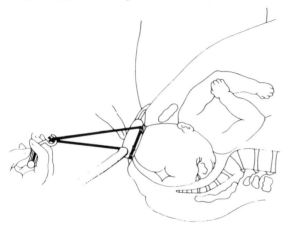

Fig. 5.47(b)   Anterior rotation with slightly downward traction, the thumb acting as a pivot point

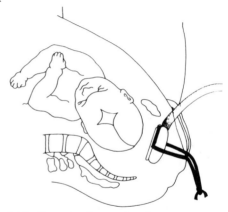

Fig. 5.49   Insertion into perineal space is performed in one movement

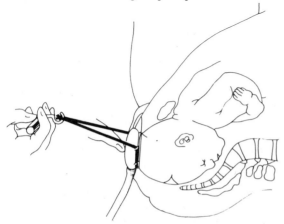

Fig. 5.47(c)   Anterior rotation is completed

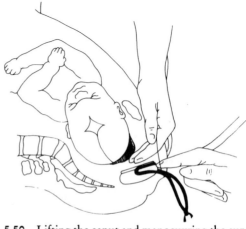

Fig. 5.50   Lifting the caput and manoeuvring the cup over the flexion point

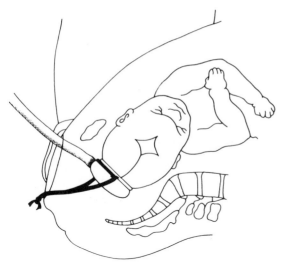

Fig. 5.51 Checking that the application is correct

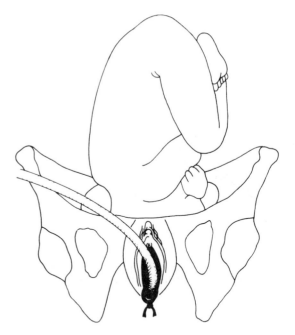

Fig. 5.52(b) The operator's view

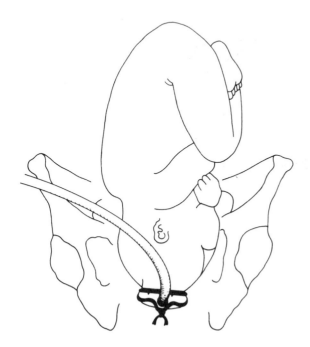

Fig. 5.52(a) Correct application

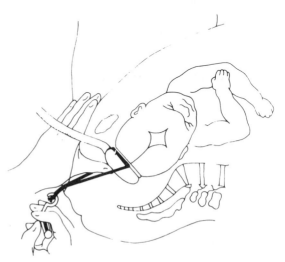

Fig. 5.53 Thumb counterpressure with initial pull while directing traction towards the floor

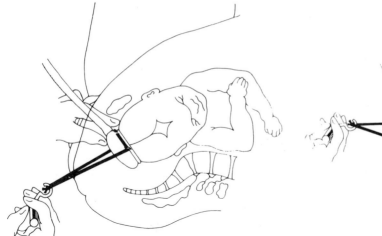

Fig. 5.54   Synclitism of the head causes lengthening of the cord and enables the finger-thumb position to be adopted

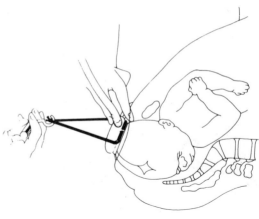

Fig. 5.56   Autorotation occurring during descent

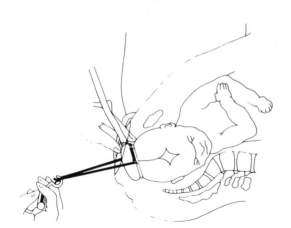

Fig. 5.55   Descent to the level of the pelvic floor

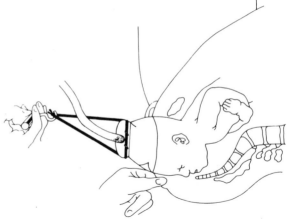

Fig. 5.57   Delivering the head

6

EFFICIENCY OF VACUUM EXTRACTION

DIFFICULT OR FAILED VACUUM EXTRACTION

There are two basic reasons why vacuum extraction may be difficult or may not succeed: either the head fails to descend or descends too slowly; or detachment of the cup occurs and results in the procedure being abandoned. Cephalopelvic disproportion must always be considered when difficulty is encountered during vacuum extraction, and every effort should be made to exclude it before proceeding with the delivery in order to avoid injuring the fetus[2]. True disproportion,

however, is uncommon and the cause of the difficulty is more likely to be either incorrect technique or relative disproportion that is disproportion associated with malpositions of the fetal occiput and deflexion and asynclitism of the head[31, 87]. Correct application of the vacuum cup, by promoting flexion and synclitism, should reduce the size of the presenting diameters and help to make the delivery easier. In addition, traction directed in the line of the axis of the birth canal should assist the head to descend with the least resistance. For mid pelvic procedures, this is generally in a more posterior direction (towards the sacrum).

Table 6.1 Failed vacuum extraction – rigid cups

Author	Number	Number failed	%	Type of cup
Bird[25]	2452	13	(0.5)	Bird Anterior and Posterior
Broekhuizen[88]	256	10	(4)	Bird Anterior
Carmody[71]	60	4	(7)	Bird original
Carmody[71]	55	4	(7)	Bird New Generation
Chuckwudebelu[89]	225	21	(14)	Malmstrom
Cohn[78]	127	13	(11)	Malmstrom and Bird
Ehlers[90]	107	13	(12)	Malmstrom
Hammarstrom[77]	50	1	(2)	Malmstrom
Hofmeyr[79]	18	0	(0)	Bird Anterior and O'Neil
Lasbrey[19]	121	12	(10)	Malmstrom
Moolgaoker[66]	86	47	(55)	Malmstrom
Nyirjesy[91]	109	14	(13)	Malmstrom
Punnonen[92]	223	15	(7)	Malmstrom
Schenker[93]	300	20	(7)	Malmstrom
Thiery[69]	210	1	(0.5)	Malmstrom
Thiery[69]	200	6	(3)	O'Neil
Vacca[39]	142	19	(13)	Bird Anterior and Posterior
TOTAL	**4741**	**213**	**(4.5)**	

Table 6.2 Failed vacuum extraction – soft cups

Author	Number	Number failed	%	Type of cup
Cohn[78]	127	21	(16)	Silc
Dell[72]	36	10	(28)	Silastic
Dell[72]	37	4	(11)	Mityvac
Hammarstrom[77]	50	9	(18)	Silastic
Hastie[75]	100	54	(54)	Silastic
Hofmeyr[79]	13	3	(23)	Silc and Silastic
Johanson[38]	127	27	(22)	Silc
Maryniak[94]	431	12	(10)	Silastic
Svigos[76]	153	10	(7)	Silastic
TOTAL	1074	150	(14)	

In the published studies displayed in Tables 6.1 (metal cups) and 6.2 (soft cups), the mean failure rate for the metal cups was 4.5 per cent and for the soft cups 14 per cent, although the range in both groups varied widely. Evidence from the Oxford Database of Perinatal Trials also indicates that soft vacuum extractor cups are significantly more likely to fail to achieve vaginal delivery than metal cups[14]. Failure was more frequent when the station of the head was high (above the ischial spines)[25, 42], when the procedure was attempted before full dilatation of the cervix[66, 78, 91] and where the occiput was lateral or posterior[19, 75, 76, 77, 78, 79]. Bird has defined the ideal (flexing median) application site[9] and demonstrated that good results with the vacuum extractor depended, to a large extent, on correct applications of the cup. The relationship between application of the cup and failure rate is shown in Table 6.3 which displays data derived from an observational study of 244 rotational vacuum extractions. In the group with flexing

median applications, only 4 per cent of the vacuum extractions were unsuccessful compared with 35 per cent where the applications were deflexing and paramedian. Of the 363 mothers who had unsuccessful vacuum extractions in the studies reported in Tables 6.1 and 6.2, 82 per cent subsequently had assisted vaginal deliveries, usually with the aid of forceps. This suggests that incorrect technique with the vacuum extractor, rather than cephalo-pelvic disproportion, was responsible for failure of the procedure. Although few would disagree that posterior and lateral positions of the occiput make vacuum extraction more difficult, careful technique particularly paying attention to achieving a flexing median application should substantially reduce the number of failed procedures.

Table 6.3 The effect of cup application in OL and OP positions – failure to deliver

Application of cup	Number	Failed vacuum Number	%
Flexing	151	12	8
– median	– 103	– 4	– 4
– paramedian	– 48	– 8	– 17
Deflexing	93	30	32
– median	– 38	– 11	– 29
– paramedian	– 55	– 19	– 35
TOTAL	244	42	17

DETACHMENT OF THE CUP

Studies that reported detachment of the cup are shown in Tables 6.4 (metal cups) and 6.5 (soft cups). Detachment occurred in 14 per cent of the vacuum extractions using metal cups and in 34 per cent of the procedures using soft cups. Such high detachment rates, especially with the soft cups, should not be accepted without trying to identify an explanation of the possible causes because they may reflect either problems with the instrument or with the way the instrument is used. Furthermore, injury to the fetal scalp is associated with sudden detachment of the cup[25, 72, 95] and, although it is usually superficial and minor, it is likely to be more serious if the detachment occurs after the cup has been subjected to strong traction.

Cup detachment may occur for the following reasons: incorrect traction technique, deflexing or

Table 6.4 Detachment – rigid cups

Author	Number	Number detached	%	Type of cup
Carmody[71]	60	4	(7)	Bird original
Carmody[71]	55	9	(16)	Bird New Generation
Cohn[78]	127	10	(8)	Malmstrom and Bird
Hofmeyr[79]	18	7	(39)	Bird and O'Neil
Nyirjesy[91]	109	24	(22)	Malmstrom
Punnonen[92]	223	42	(19)	Malmstrom
Thiery[69]	210	27	(13)	Malmstrom
Thiery[69]	200	18	(9)	O'Neil
TOTAL	1002	141	14	

Table 6.5 Detachment – soft cups

Author	Number	Number detached	%	Type of cup
Cohn[78]	127	25	(20)	Silc
Dell[72]	36	10	(28)	Silastic
Dell[72]	37	13	(35)	Mityvac
Hastie[75]	100	50	(50)	Silastic
Hofmeyr[79]	13	6	(46)	Silc and Silastic
Johanson[38]	127	44	(35)	Silc
TOTAL	440	148	(34)	

paramedian application, a large caput succedaneum; maternal tissue or scalp electrode caught under the cup; inadequate vacuum pressure or faulty equipment. Attachment of the cup is most effective when the direction of traction is perpendicular to the cup. Oblique traction on the other hand by lifting one edge of the cup and depressing the other predisposes to cup detachment. Pulling too hard, in the wrong direction or when uterine contractions are weak may also dislodge the cup. For the same reason, as soon as the mother ceases to push, the operator should relax the traction. Resistance to descent of the head is increased in malpositions that are associated with some degree of extension (less than complete flexion) and asynclitism. With deflexing and paramedian applications correction of malposition is unlikely to occur, with the result that the procedure is rendered more difficult. If the traction force required to overcome resistance to descent is greater than the adhesive force of the cup, detachment will occur. A paramedian application combined with oblique traction is a common cause of cup detachment. Unlike median applications where the scalp base under the cup extends well beyond the margins to form an airtight seal (Fig. 6.1), paramedian applications have the scalp on one side of the head 'falling away' from the edge of the cup making an effective seal difficult to maintain when traction is applied. Detachment of the cup with weak traction occurs more readily when the cup is applied over a large caput succedaneum and the direction of traction is oblique. Other causes are loss of pressure or faulty vacuum apparatus, or maternal tissue or scalp electrode caught under the cup. Regular maintenance of the equipment and careful technique will avoid these minor complications. Correct application of the cup and traction in the axis of the birth canal should reduce the number of detachments from other causes. Complete detachment may be prevented by exerting counterpressure on the cup with the finger-thumb technique during traction and by ceasing to pull when the contraction passes and the mother stops pushing.

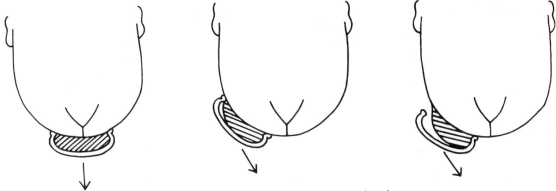

Fig. 6.1   Paramedian applications and oblique traction predispose to cup detachment

INTERNAL ROTATION

The wide variation in reported anterior rotation rates from lateral and posterior positions of the occiput, shown in Table 6.6, has caused some obstetricians to question the value of the vacuum extractor as a rotator of the malpositioned head. Whether rotation occurs in an anterior or posterior direction during vacuum extraction is sometimes considered to be a function of the shape and size of the fetal head and of the maternal pelvis, but Bird[9] has shown that failure of anterior rotation in occipitoposterior and lateral positions is almost always the result of incorrect applications of the cup and seldom the result of pelvic shape. This association between anterior rotation of the occiput and application of the cup is demonstrated in Table 6.7. In 244 vacuum extractions attempted where the occiput was lateral or posterior, rotation occurred overall in 68 per cent; however, in the group where cup application was flexing, rotation occurred in 94 per cent compared with only 27 per cent where the application was deflexing.

Epidural analgesia may predispose to malposition of the head by interfering with the normal tone of the muscles of the pelvic floor[96] but this suggestion has been disputed[97, 98]. Anterior rotation from occipitoposterior and lateral positions will usually occur spontaneously during vacuum extraction provided the application of the cup causes flexion[9]. This auto-rotation should occur without any assistance from the obstetrician[99], and any attempt to assist rotation by manipulation of the cup may lead to the cup slipping on the scalp[2, 100]. The operator may observe that internal rotation is occurring by noting the relative position of the suction tubing where it joins the cup (Fig. 6.2); as the head rotates the tubing will be seen to move in the corresponding clockwise or anti-clockwise direction. Failed anterior rotations, like difficult or failed vacuum extractions, are often the result of incorrect applications of the cup which promote or fail to correct deflexion and asynclitism. Traction and compression forces exerted on the fetal head are greater when delivery occurs in the occipitoposterior position[86], and the

Table 6.6   Anterior rotation in OL/OP positions

Author	Number of OL/OP	Rotation to OA		Type of cup
		Number	%	
Bird[9]	100	94	(94)	Bird Posterior
Chukwudubelu[89]	80	58	(73)	Malmstrom
Johanson[38]	52	36	(69)	Silc
Moolgaoker[66]	74	37	(50)	Malmstrom
Vacca[39]	244	166	(68)	Malmstrom and Bird
TOTAL	550	391	(72)	

Table 6.7 The effect of cup application in OL and OP positions – anterior rotation

Application of cup	Number	Anterior rotation	
		Number	%
Flexing	151	142	94
– median	– 103	– 99	– 96
– paramedian	– 48	– 43	– 90
Deflexing	93	25	27
– median	– 38	– 9	– 24
– paramedian	– 55	– 16	– 29
TOTAL	**244**	**167**	**68**

likelihood of failed vacuum extraction, injury to the perineum and injury to the fetus may be increased in face-to-pubis delivery[9, 66]. If the application of the cup is flexing median, anterior rotation can be expected to occur in about 95 per cent of extractions when the occiput is lateral or posterior[25].

DURATION OF THE PROCEDURE

One criticism of vacuum extraction is that the procedure takes too long in some circumstances and forceps delivery may be preferred because it is perceived to be quicker. One reason that may contribute to this belief is the long-standing but incorrect recommendation that up to ten minutes be allowed to form the chignon[24], even though it has been demonstrated that an adequate chignon is formed after two minutes of applying the vacuum[18, 101] and that traction may be started after this shorter time interval. For most vacuum extractions, adequate analgesia is provided by perineal infiltration with local anaesthetic agents and time need not be spent instituting the more complex forms of pain relief that are often required for forceps delivery.

Furthermore, considerable time will be saved if the vacuum cup and tubing are pre-assembled in a transparent sterile plastic packet and if the pump is properly maintained and ready for immediate use. Although the time from application of the instrument to the delivery may favour the forceps, evidence from randomized controlled comparisons of vacuum extraction and forceps delivery suggests that the average time interval from the decision to deliver the baby to the actual delivery is similar for both instruments[38, 39].

COMPRESSION AND TRACTION FORCES

For the fetal head to pass through the birth canal, the powers exerted on it must be greater than the sum of the resisting forces in the pelvis. The powers may be enhanced by increasing the propulsive forces (uterine contractions, maternal expulsive effort); by reducing the resisting forces (decreasing the size of the presenting diameters of the fetal head) so that existing powers are rendered more effective; or by applying traction to the fetal

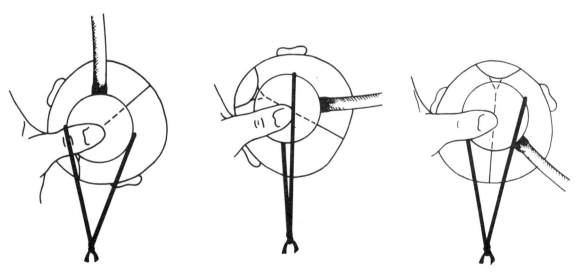

Fig. 6.2 Observing autorotation by the change in position of the suction tube

head (vacuum extraction). In normal labour, compression force acting on the head depends on the friction between the maternal tissues, the size of the presenting diameters of the head, and the strength of the expulsive powers. Forces are modified by the pliable nature of the scalp bones which allows the head to reduce its dimensions in one plane and increase them in another, and by rotation and flexion of the fetal head as an adaptation to the curved birth canal. Resistance to delivery is least when the largest diameters of the head meet the widest diameters of the pelvis at any given level in the birth canal.

Many investigators have tried to define what forces constitute safe levels of traction and compression. The upper limits of safety are not known but a traction force of 23 kgms has been suggested[102]. During the expulsive phase of the second stage of spontaneous labour, forces acting on the fetal head have been calculated to be between 8.4 kgms[86] and 15 kgms[23]. The amount of traction force which the vacuum cup will accept before it comes off the scalp depends mainly on the shape, diameter and depth of the cup, the level of negative pressure in the cup and the direction of the applied force[25]. Saling observed that a 60 mm Malmstrom cup withstood a traction force of 20 kgms and that detachment did not occur if the force was less than 20 kgms[103]. Moolgaoker, using electronic measurement equipment, found that a 50 mm Malmstrom cup with a negative pressure of 0.8 kgms/cm^2 accepted pulls of up to 21.8 kgms[102]. Bird tested his original modification of the Malmstrom cup on an artificial scalp and found that it withstood a pull of 11.3 kgms when traction was applied perpendicular to the 50 mm cup and 5.8 kgms when the direction of traction was oblique at 45 degrees to the perpendicular[4]. In a laboratory setting, Duchon found that the maximum traction forces before cup detachment occurred were 13, 20 and 18 kgms for the 50 mm Bird, the Silastic and the Mytivac cups respectively and that the maximum traction force was greater with increasing negative pressure and with increasing cup size[104]. Hofmeyr compared rigid and soft vacuum extractor cups in a randomized controlled trial, and concluded that greater traction forces could be generated using the rigid cups[79].

Malmstrom contended that when the cup is applied correctly to the head, traction force acts at the attachment of the scalp to the frontal, temporal and occipital ridges at the base of the skull[5]. He claimed that traction with the vacuum extractor did not cause any significant compression on the fetal head because the forces applied to the scalp were distributed over the whole surface of the presenting part. The force which might compress the sides of the fetal head appeared to be counterbalanced during traction by pressure on the inside of the skull. Issel maintained that with traction forces of less than 20 kgms, compression forces of between 1 and 4 kgms were active but increased rapidly with traction forces greater than 20 kgms[105]. Other investigators believed that distortion of the fetal skull must take place when traction is applied causing the head to become elongated in the direction of pull and flattened from side to side. If traction is excessive, there may then be a risk of rupture of the sagittal sinus or tearing of the falx at its attachment to the tentorium, and the sudden jumping apart of the parietal bones when the cup pulls off may cause contusion to the underlying brain substance[105, 106]. Recording the maximum traction or compression force at a single point may not be the most appropriate measure since total forces acting on the fetus depend on the length of time such a force is exerted, how rapidly a peak is reached, and on the number of tractions[102, 107]. Assumptions that compression of the head was directly proportional to the traction applied were not confirmed except in the occipitoposterior position, where compression force did parallel traction force.

Ultimately it is the operator who decides how much extra force, in addition to the normal compression forces of labour, will be exerted on the fetal head as a result of vacuum extraction. The difference between excessive, average or minimum force in delivery may depend primarily on the attending obstetrician's knowledge of how to correct abnormalities and to deliver along the path of least resistance[86]. The least additional force to effect delivery with vacuum extraction will result from flexing median applications of the cup, followed by traction in the line of the axis of the birth canal. Total force will be reduced if a limit is placed on the duration of the procedure and on the number of pulls.

7

EFFECTS OF VACUUM EXTRACTION

EFFECTS OF VACUUM EXTRACTION ON THE MOTHER

Injury to the genital tract

Early studies comparing vacuum extraction with forceps delivery suggested that less injury to the birth canal was associated with the vacuum extractor[33, 93, 99]. Evidence from randomized controlled comparisons of vacuum and forceps delivery [19, 26, 38, 72] has confirmed that the vacuum extractor is the safer instrument for the mother. Maternal injury has been reported following vacuum extraction but usually it has occurred in mothers with predisposing factors such as previous caesarean section, obstructed labour, high fetal head, incompletely dilated cervix or when failure of the procedure has been followed by attempted forceps delivery[39, 66, 91, 108, 109]. Of the 363 mothers who had failed vacuum extractions in the studies shown in Tables 6.1 and 6.2 (pp. 63 and 64), 70 per cent subsequently had vaginal deliveries completed with forceps and some others who had caesarean deliveries also had prior attempts with forceps that were unsuccessful. This predisposing factor is sometimes overlooked when adverse outcomes are attributed to the vacuum extractor[66, 75]. If the vacuum extractor is used correctly, the incidence of maternal injury should be low and not greater than that occurring after spontaneous delivery because the cup does not encroach on the upper genital tract nor does it come between the presenting part and the wall of the birth canal.

Maternal analgesia

Almost all vacuum extractions may be performed with relatively simple forms of analgesia. Perineal infiltration with local anaesthetic agents usually suffices for all types of extractions including rotational procedures although some operators prefer pudendal nerve block[38, 39]. General and regional anaesthesia is more likely to be used if instrumental vaginal delivery is attempted with forceps than with the vacuum extractor[110]. Epidural analgesia should not be instituted for the purposes of vacuum extraction but some mothers will have received this form of pain relief in the first stage of labour. In these mothers, operators will be required to adjust their technique to compensate for the loss of bearing down sensation in order to avoid using additional traction force to overcome any reduction in maternal expulsive power. The fact that general anaesthesia is not necessary[2], and indeed may be regarded as a contraindication, helps to make vacuum extraction a safer procedure for the mother.

Mothers' views

Women who had participated in randomized controlled trials of forceps and vacuum extraction[38, 65] were questioned about their experiences of the two methods of assisted delivery. Mothers who were randomly allocated to vacuum extraction reported less discomfort during[65] and following[38] delivery. This may have been attributable to the fact that there were fewer significant injuries in mothers delivered by this method. On the other hand, women allocated to vacuum extraction had more worries about their babies. They voiced concern about the baby's appearance, possibly due to the presence of a chignon or cup marking and the development of mild neonatal jaundice. They were reassured, however, from the explanations given by the medical and nursing staff when they expressed their concerns. Babies who were born during one of the randomized trials comparing forceps and vacuum extraction[39] were reassessed at nine months of age[111]. Parental worries were not only rare but were equally distributed between the two groups and appeared to be unrelated to the method of delivery.

EFFECTS OF VACUUM EXTRACTION ON THE INFANT

Fetal hypoxia and neonatal condition

Neonatal behaviour and irritability after vacuum extraction may be related to the infant's condition *in utero*[76] and to the indication for delivery[112], as well as to the way the instrument is used. Neonatal depression after clinically indicated vacuum extraction has been found to be related to the degree of difficulty of the procedure[103]. Hypoxia was not associated with vacuum extraction performed for outlet delivery or when the duration of the second stage of labour was not prolonged[103], nor with easy extractions completed with no more than four pulls[114, 115]. Most behavioural disturbances were transient and no longer detectable a few days after birth[4, 32]. Opinion is divided, however, on the question of whether elective vacuum extraction causes more[116] or less[117] neonatal depression than spontaneous delivery. In randomized studies comparing the condition of babies delivered by forceps or vacuum extraction, no significant differences were found in Apgar scores, in rates of endotracheal intubation, in the time taken to establish regular respirations or in admission rates to special care baby units[38, 39, 72].

Retinal haemorrhage

Although retinal haemorrhages occur in infants following normal birth, they are more common after instrumental delivery[118]. The mechanism responsible for their appearance is still unknown but the low incidence in babies born by caesarean section suggests that forces associated with the passage of the fetal head through the birth canal predispose to the lesion. Retinal haemorrhages have been found to be associated with paramedian

applications of the cup[119] and with the degree of difficulty of the procedure[120, 121]. Several authors have reported more retinal haemorrhages following vacuum extraction than after forceps delivery[90, 118, 122], but others were not able to confirm such differences[38, 123]. Evidence from randomized trials suggests that vacuum extraction is associated with more retinal haemorrhages than forceps delivery[110] (Knuppel. R. 1991, personal communication). The clinical significance of retinal haemorrhages is unclear as they appear to be transient lesions leaving no residual ill effects. The suggestion that bleeding into the retina may be associated with subclinical cerebral trauma[122] could not be substantiated by correlating the haemorrhages with neurobehaviour of infants after birth[124] nor could any association be established between the ocular findings at birth and later childhood visual development[119]

Chignon, scalp marking and abrasion

The chignon or artificial caput succedaneum is a swelling of the scalp that develops inside the cup when the vacuum is induced and is the means by which the cup adheres to the scalp. The chignon is most obvious immediately following removal of the cup from the scalp but it rapidly decreases in size to become a diffuse swelling within one hour of birth and then behaves like a normal caput succedaneum usually disappearing over one or two days. Occasionally the colour of the scalp over the chignon may be quite dark at first but this fades quickly and disappears, usually by the third day. Some marking of the baby's scalp is always present after vacuum extraction but the extent to which it is visible will depend on the amount of hair present on the scalp. Such markings disappear after a few days[24] and are without clinical significance[72]. Abrasions to the scalp may occur with vacuum extraction, the reported incidence ranging from 0.8 per cent to 82 per cent[77, 95]. The majority are superficial and small in size but occasionally may be large and cosmetically unsightly. Difficult vacuum extractions with prolonged traction and sudden cup detachments predispose to injuries of the scalp[25, 72, 95]. Abrasions most often occur along the edge of the cup that is nearer the side of the baby's head and are commonly seen in association with paramedian applications. Thus, the number of abrasions may be reduced with correct application of the cup, avoiding prolonged traction and preventing cup detachment. Although complications to abrasions have been reported[125], they are rare and the lesions nearly always heal rapidly leaving no traces[2]. The injured area should be kept clean with antiseptic solution and treated with topical antibiotic ointment until a scab develops. During the procedure, parents should be informed of the appearance of a chignon and if superficial injury to the scalp occurs, be reassured as soon as possible after the delivery[23, 42, 65]. Regular inspections of the baby should be carried out in the presence of the mother during the postnatal period and follow-up arrangements made if the lesions have not healed prior to the infant's discharge from hospital.

Cephalhaematoma and subcutaneous haematoma

Cephalhaematomas are collections of blood that accumulate under the periosteum of the skull bones, usually the parietal, and are characteristically limited to the confines of the cranial bone (Fig. 7.1.) They should be distinguished from subcutaneous (cup) haematomas which are small collections of blood under the skin at the site of application of the cup and which are not always limited by the suture lines[95]. Reported incidences for cephalhaematomas range from 1 per cent to 26 per cent with a mean incidence of 6 per cent[78, 95]. The wide variation in incidence may be partly explained by the fact that they sometimes develop several hours after delivery[72] and also because small haematomas may pass unnoticed. Cephalhaematomas occur more frequently after vacuum extraction than after forceps[16, 39, 110, 123, 126] or spontaneous[2, 127] delivery. Bleeding from the scalp and cephalhaematoma formation have been described with vacuum extraction after fetal blood sampling[37], but no complications of this nature

were reported in other studies[38, 39, 40]. Resolution of subcutaneous haematomas occurs rapidly over a matter of days but cephalhaematomas may take longer, possibly a few weeks to disappear[72]. Complications are rare and no specific therapy is required other than reassurance of the parents.

Subgaleal (subaponeurotic) haemorrhage

A subgaleal haematoma is formed when bleeding occurs into the potential space beneath the aponeurosis of the scalp (Fig. 7.2). It may be a life-threatening condition for the newborn baby and is the most serious complication associated with vacuum extraction[128]. The danger arises because the subaponeurotic space stretches over the whole of the cranial vault, and a large proportion of the baby's blood volume may accumulate in this space from damage to emissary veins[74]. Although subgaleal haemorrhage may occur after forceps and spontaneous deliveries[129], the incidence has increased considerably since the introduction of the vacuum extractor into obstetric practice[25, 130]. Reported incidences of subgaleal haemorrhage in earlier studies have been between 1 per cent and 3.8 per cent of all vacuum extractions[2] but have been much less common in more recent surveys[39, 72, 78, 126]. Subgaleal haemorrhage is almost always preceded by difficult extraction and is more likely to occur if fetal hypoxia or coagulopathy are present[131].

Traction that does not cause descent of the head (negative traction)[25] may pull the aponeurosis from the cranium and injure the underlying veins. Immediately after delivery, the scalp in these babies has a characteristic loose feel and moves freely over the underlying bones when palpated. All babies' heads should be carefully examined

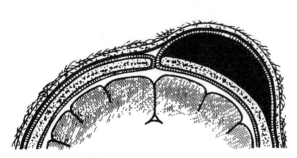

Fig. 7.1   Cephalhaematoma

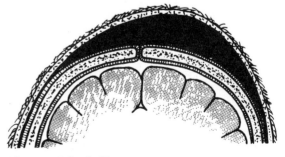

Fig. 7.2   Subgaleal haematoma

after vacuum extraction and re-examined at regular intervals if the extraction was difficult.

Haemorrhage into the subgaleal space may occur over several hours following delivery and unless careful observations are made, the bleeding may not become obvious until the haematoma is extensive. At this stage, there may be a fluctuant or diffuse swelling under the scalp which may be indented with finger pressure. The baby may show signs of circulatory collapse with pallor, hypotension, raised pulse rate and a fall in haematocrit. Early and prompt recognition of subaponeurotic bleeding, careful monitoring of the baby's condition and coagulation status, use of a pressure bandage to the scalp and early transfusion with blood or colloid should reduce morbidity and prevent mortality from this condition[128]. The volume of blood or colloid required for transfusion in a neonate with subgaleal haemorrhage may be calculated by allowing 38 mls for each centimetre by which the head circumference exceeds the 50th centile for that baby[129]. If consumptive coagulopathy is present, the baby should be transfused with fresh frozen plasma or fresh whole blood. Avoiding difficult vacuum extractions and prolonged traction is a simple and effective method of preventing subgaleal haemorrhage.

Neonatal jaundice

Although jaundice has been reported to be more common after vacuum extraction than after forceps or spontaneous delivery[132, 133], other observers have found no differences in the incidence[2, 42, 126]. The clinical assessment of jaundice may be very inaccurate as is demonstrated when the serum bilirubin levels of jaundiced babies are compared with the clinical diagnoses[78]. In a randomized controlled study where bilirubin levels were performed, no significant differences in the incidence of hyperbilirubinaemia or in the number of babies requiring phototherapy were found, although the numbers in the study were small[39]. In another randomized study, clinically apparent jaundice was more common in the vacuum extraction group but this did not have clinical significance as there was no difference in treatment[39]. Evidence from the Oxford Database of Perinatal Trials suggests that jaundice is more common after vacuum extraction but that there is no difference in the number of babies requiring phototherapy[110].

Intracranial haemorrhage

Modern imaging techniques have revealed that intracranial haemorrhage in the term newborn infant is more common than was previously realized[134]. While difficult vacuum extractions may produce scalp trauma, serious intracranial injury is rare[95] and depends to a large extent on the way the instrument is used[112, 135].

Subdural bleeding from injury to intracranial veins has been reported following difficult operative delivery[136] in high-risk obstetric patients[19, 35]. Intracranial compartments of the brain are separated vertically by the falx cerebri and horizontally by the tentorium cerebelli (Fig. 7.3). These supporting structures are accompanied by thin walled venous sinuses which under normal circumstances, can withstand the moulding and compression of labour and delivery. However, damage to the falx or tentorium and to their venous sinuses may occur when compression on the head is excessive as may happen when vacuum extraction is attempted in the presence of severe moulding. By carefully assessing the level of the head and degree of moulding, by achieving correct applications of the cup and by limiting the number of pulls[19], the risk of intracranial injury should be minimal.

Clinical manifestations of intracranial bleeding are variable but babies almost always show abnormal neurological signs such as increasing irritability, neonatal depression, apnoea or convulsions[137]. Intracranial haemorrhage should always be considered in the differential diagnosis if the baby exhibits abnormal neonatal behaviour after difficult vacuum extraction so that early diagnosis may lead promptly to more effective treatment[138].

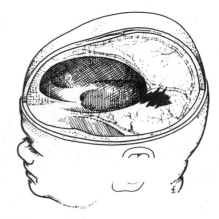

Fig. 7.3 Intracranial haematoma

Shoulder dystocia

Shoulder dystocia is an obstetric emergency that may cause fetal death or a number of serious injuries which include brachial plexus damage, fractures of the clavicle and humerus, facial trauma and birth asphyxia. This complication has been estimated to occur in about 3 per 1000 of all cephalic vaginal births[139, 140] but the incidence rises as the fetal size increases. About 3 per cent of infants weighing more than 4 kgms at birth will be subjected to some difficulty with the delivery of the shoulders but the risk is greater if the second stage of labour is complicated by slow progress or delay and failure of descent of the head[141].

A recommendation has been proposed for a selective policy of caesarean section for women in whom the fetal weight was estimated to be above 4000 grams and where there was abnormal progress in labour[141]. However, since the incidence of birth trauma in infants weighing over 4000 grams with shoulder dystocia in the study was 12.7 per cent, it was calculated that 200 caesarean sections would be required in women with macrosomic infants to prevent three cases of birth trauma[142]. Furthermore, since almost half of the infants who developed shoulder dystocia weighed less than 4000 grams[143] and even if fetal weight estimation were accurate, such a policy would have prevented only 11 per cent of possible cases of shoulder dystocia, while 68 per cent of the operations would have been unnecessary[144].

There is at present no reliable method of antenatal prediction of shoulder dystocia[145, 146]. Clinical estimation of fetal size can be notoriously inaccurate and only a minority of infants with clinical predisposing factors or labour abnormalities will develop the complication. Comparing the measurements of the fetal transthoracic and biparietal diameters obtained by ultrasonography has been suggested as a method of improving the prediction rate[147] but only six of sixteen infants weighing more than 4000 grams were able to be identified prior to delivery despite having had serial ultrasonography from 28 weeks onwards[148]. In a case control study of shoulder dystocia, high birthweight was confirmed to be a significant factor regardless of which method of delivery was used[146]. When birthweight was controlled in the analysis, midforceps and midcavity vacuum extraction remained significantly associated with brachial nerve injury. The authors concluded that with the current limitations in predicting birthweight accurately, the only risk factor that may be avoided is mid pelvic instrumental delivery. The findings also suggested that the vacuum extractor was being used to substitute the forceps in mid pelvic instrumental procedures, a practice that may allow an attendant with less technical skill and possibly less experience in judgment to attempt deliveries previously included in the midforceps category. Shoulder dystocia appears to be more common with extractors when the cup is applied before the cervix is fully dilated.

Prevention of shoulder dystocia by prophylactic use of caesarean section for all patients with risk factors does not appear to be practical or advisable[149]. Because the majority of infants who will experience shoulder dystocia cannot be identified before labour, all birth attendants should be skilled in the management of this complication and be on the alert for its unexpected development. Many management protocols have been suggested for shoulder dystocia[150], ranging from relatively simple manipulations to more complex manoeuvres. The attendant, however, should have formulated a definite plan of action[149, 151, 152] and should proceed in a predetermined fashion if serious injury to the infant and mother from this condition is to be avoided or reduced to a minimum.

Perinatal mortality

In a comprehensive review of vacuum extraction[95], the uncorrected perinatal mortality rate was 25.8 per 1000 vacuum extractions, and 15.5 per 1000 extractions when corrected for fetal anomaly and intrauterine death. Death occurring from cranial and intracranial injuries possibly resulting from the method of delivery was estimated to be 2 per 1000 vacuum extractions. Most of these reports were published in the early years of vacuum extraction[25] when the instrument was commonly used in circumstances not generally recommended by most modern operators. In recent controlled studies[26, 38, 69, 71], perinatal deaths were rare and not attributable to the vacuum extractor[39, 78].

Long term effects

Conclusions drawn from retrospective studies about long term sequelae of instrumental delivery for the neonate may be misleading due to a lack of adequate controls[153, 154]. At present, there is not enough information available to assess the effects of vacuum extraction on the long term condition of the infants[26]. In a review of follow-up studies of cohorts of babies born after operative vaginal delivery, intellectual impairment or cerebral palsies were rarely seen except when birth trauma was combined with birth asphyxia[155]. The long term development of a group of babies born by vacuum extraction and a group born spontaneously was compared in one study at 14 months of age[156], and in another at 14 years of age[112] and no differences were found in either study. No significant differences were found when babies who had been born during a randomized trial comparing forceps and vacuum extration[39] were reassessed at 9 months of age[111], nor in another controlled study with follow-up data to six months of age[72].

8

SAFETY MEASURES AND TRAINING

SAFETY MEASURES

Safety of vacuum extraction depends on careful consideration of a number of factors, several of which may be evaluated before the procedure, many during the procedure itself and a few after vacuum extraction is completed.

Before vacuum extraction

Fetal distress as the primary or associated indication for vacuum extraction must be monitored carefully to ensure that additional stress from the procedure does not exceed recommended safety limits. Since outcome may be predetermined by the condition of the fetus *in utero*, caesarean section may be the safer option for delivery if fetal distress is more than mild. Indications for vacuum extraction should be separated into standard and special categories, as is suggested in Table 3.1 (see p. 29). In general, procedures in the standard group have a wider margin of safety than those in the special group. Special uses of the vacuum extractor will be contraindications for all but the most experienced operators. Because of the risks to the fetus and mother, vacuum extraction should not be attempted before the cervix is fully dilated. There may be a few exceptions to this rule in special circumstances, but only if strict criteria are followed.

Outcome with the vacuum extractor is closely related to the selection of suitable patients which, in practice, may be made by considering the station of the presenting part, the degree of moulding and the position of the fetal head (see Table 3.2 on p. 36). When the head is visible at the outlet of the pelvis or is stationed on the pelvic floor, the procedure is easily performed and the risks to the fetus are minimal. On the other hand, mid-pelvic extractions demand a high level of technical skill as well as training in rotational vacuum extraction.

If labour is complicated by delay in the second stage and the size of the fetus is estimated to be large, the possibility of a difficult extraction should be anticipated. Shoulder dystocia is also more common when this combination of factors is present. For these reasons, if the operator is not sufficiently experienced or has not been trained in the method of rotational vacuum extraction, caesarean section is the safer method of delivery for the fetus.

Vacuum extraction should not be attempted if cephalopelvic disproportion is present, or when the station of the fetal head is high; the practice of applying a vacuum cup to the head in order to bring the presenting part down to a lower station so that delivery may be completed with forceps should be discouraged.

During vacuum extraction

The importance of a correct application of the vacuum cup as a factor exercising a major influence on outcome cannot be overemphasized. Correct application of the cup depends on knowledge of the flexion point and the operator's ability to apply the cup over the ideal site on the fetal head. For malpositions, the choice of cup should be one that includes the posterior design principle that allows correct application to the head when the flexion point is not readily accessible.

The amount of traction force required to deliver the baby will be inversely proportional to the maternal expulsive effort. For this reason, the operator should ensure that uterine contractions and maternal expulsive powers are effective. Oxytocin should be administered by intravenous infusion to enhance contractions if there is a suspicion of hypotonic uterine action. If epidural analgesia has been administered, the operator should compensate for the absence of the mother's desire to bear down by informing her when she is pushing correctly and encouraging her to maximum effort at the appropriate time. General anaesthesia, which abolishes the voluntary powers and diminishes uterine contractions, should not be used for vacuum extraction because greater reliance is placed on traction for delivery, and as a consequence the risk of fetal injury is increased. If voluntary expulsive effort is reduced, the obstetrician may find it helpful to spend a little time gaining the mother's confidence and cooperation by explaining the reasons for the procedure and the need for her active involvement in the birth.

Traction should be applied only during a contraction in conjunction with the mother's expulsive efforts. As soon as the contraction passes or the mother stops pushing, traction should cease. The head, not just the scalp, must begin to move with the first pull and descent must occur with each subsequent pull. In most cases, delivery may be completed or almost completed in three pulls. If epidural analgesia has been administered, however, one or two gentle pulls may help the mother to become accustomed to pushing effectively in the absence of a bearing down sensation. Pulls that do not cause the head to descend (negative pulls) must be differentiated from those that do, as they are more likely to cause subgaleal haemorrhage. The finger-thumb position of the non-pulling hand should be maintained until the head has crowned because it serves to inform the operator that the head, and not just the scalp, is descending with traction. It also helps to prevent complete detachment of the cup.

Cup detachment should not be regarded as a safety mechanism of the vacuum extractor but should be seen as a warning sign of cephalopelvic disproportion or of incorrect application of the cup. If detachment occurs, the cup should be reapplied only if the operator is convinced that the cause of the detachment is not cephalopelvic disproportion. Incorrect application of the cup and pulling in the wrong direction are common causes of cup detachment.

The fetal head should be completely delivered within 15 minutes of applying the cup. If the duration of the procedure exceeds this time limit or if satisfactory descent does not occur, traction should be discontinued and the baby delivered by caesarean section. Forceps should not be applied to the fetal head if vacuum extraction fails to deliver the baby unless the head has descended to the outlet of the pelvis.

Midcavity vacuum extractions that may be anticipated to be difficult (trial of vacuum extraction) should be performed in an operating theatre that has been prepared for caesarean section. If difficulty is encountered, the procedure should be discontinued immediately and delivery completed by caesarean section.

After vacuum extraction

After all vacuum extractions, the baby's head must be carefully examined and re-examined at regular intervals for evidence of subgaleal haemorrhage if the extraction was difficult. Prompt recognition of subgaleal bleeding, use of a pressure bandage to the scalp and early blood transfusion will reduce morbidity and prevent mortality from this condition.

TRAINING PROGRAMMES

There is no doubt that the operator is a major determinant of the success or failure of instrumental delivery and that unfavourable results associated with the vacuum extractor are often caused by the user's unfamiliarity with either the instrument or the basic rules governing its use[67]. Recommendations were proposed at the start of the modern era of vacuum extraction that are still relevant:

- *acquaintance with the instrument and with the principles of its use*
- *strict adherence to recommendations*
- *a protocol for self-education by using the instrument initially for relatively easy medical procedures and avoiding complex clinical situations.*

Although many obstetricians acquire their experience in vacuum extraction through self instruction, training under the supervision of skilled users of the instrument is preferable. Use of the vacuum extractor should form a part of all obstetric training programmes but this may be difficult to implement because the number of well trained instructors is small. In many countries, specialist obstetricians have been trained only in the use of forceps and have had little or no exposure to the vacuum extractor[34]. Furthermore, the training of obstetricians to perform mid pelvic instrumental deliveries safely has become increasingly difficult[64] and current obstetric practice is likely further to discourage the use of midcavity instrumental procedures for a number of reasons[157]: there is a willingness to allow the duration of the second stage of labour to proceed beyond the traditional time limits; operative vaginal delivery may injure the baby; and caesarean section has become a relatively safe operation which is easy to perform by anyone with basic surgical skills.

Reported rates for operative vaginal delivery vary considerably around the world and between institutions and are often independent of corresponding caesarean section rates[27, 28]. Although the justification for mid pelvic instrumental delivery has been seriously questioned[157, 158, 159], a survey of institutions in North America concluded that midforceps operations were still considered important in current obstetric practice[160]. Substituting caesarean deliveries for all midcavity instrumental procedures would not be feasible or advisable; the operation carries increased risks for the mother and does not necessarily improve the outcome for the baby[161, 162]. However, to make instrumental delivery a safe alternative to caesarean section, complications that develop during labour should be assessed by an obstetrician who is both experienced in operative obstetrics and adequately trained in the method of forceps or vacuum extraction.

An essential part of a training programme in vacuum extraction should include an understanding of the basic principles governing the instrument's use, especially with regard to correct application of the cup and traction procedure. Equally important is an appreciation of the obstetric circumstances in which the vacuum extractor may or may not be used safely. Operators who are not familiar with the vacuum extractor, whatever their seniority or skill with the forceps, should begin with a programme of straightforward outlet procedures, graduating to mid pelvic non-rotational operations and only after mastering the technique in these circumstances consider attempting the more complex rotational procedures. It is inadvisable to use the forceps for straightforward deliveries and reserve the vacuum extractor for the more challenging situations[39] because confidence and experience in the technique is best acquired by using the instrument for the easy extractions.

FORCEPS OR VACUUM EXTRACTOR?

Considerable regional and international differences exist in the preferences for forceps or vacuum extractor but the reasons for this are not clear. There are a few circumstances in which either forceps delivery or vacuum extraction is preferable[81]. For example, forceps delivery is the only alternative when assistance is required for the birth of a baby presenting by the face or for the delivery of the after-coming head in breech presentation. On the other hand, the vacuum extractor may be more suitable for the delivery of the second of twins or after symphysiotomy[62]. However, for the majority of assisted vaginal deliveries, the relative merits of forceps delivery and vacuum extraction have been the subject of considerable debate. Early comparisons of the two methods suggested that the vacuum extractor was associated with fewer maternal injuries but had more undesirable neonatal effects than the forceps and that it was less effective than the forceps for completing delivery or achieving anterior rotation in malpositions of the occiput[18, 66, 91, 102]. Such conclusions, however, should not necessarily be accepted or rejected without question as they have been derived mainly from studies using non-randomized concurrent controls and the groups of patients assigned to forceps delivery and vacuum extraction were not comparable in many important respects[163]. For example, Table 8.1 displays some differences in the cohorts of women and babies delivered by the two instruments that may have resulted in outcomes that are at variance with those derived from less biased (randomized) comparisons. Overviews (meta-analyses) of six randomized trials comparing forceps and vacuum extraction[19, 38, 39, 72, 90, 123] that have been reported in the Oxford Database of Perinatal Trials[110] have confirmed that vacuum extraction is less likely to achieve a successful vaginal delivery than forceps but, on the other hand, can be performed with less regional and general anaesthesia and is associated with less serious maternal injury.

In the newborn, cephalhaematomata have been shown to be more common with the vacuum extractor but other facial and cranial injuries were evenly distributed between the two methods. Mild

Table 8.1   Comparing vacuum extraction and forceps

Author	Vacuum extraction %	Forceps %
Broekhuizen[88]		
fetal head at or above spines	24	3
occiput posterior or lateral	59	27
Hastie[75]		
cervix not fully dilated	35	0
Moolgaoker[66]		
cervix not fully dilated	100	100
relative use of instruments	1	42
unsuccessful rotation in OL/OP	50	0
Nyirjesy[91]		
cervix not fully dilated	28	1
fetal head above spines	5	0
midcavity procedures	31	8
occiput posterior or lateral	34	7
Punnonen[92]		
fetal head at or above spines	18	6
performed by doctor in training	84	34
Schenker[93]		
cervix not fully dilated	11	0
fetal head above spines	41	0
midcavity procedures	59	27
Svigos[76]		
fetal distress	36	22
one minute Apgar <6	14	5
Wider[18]		
cervix not fully dilated	18	0
relative use of instruments	1	28

jaundice occurred more frequently in babies delivered by vacuum extraction but no significant difference was shown in the number of babies requiring phototherapy, and retinal haemorrhages were also more common after vacuum extraction although the evidence was still inconclusive.

For most indications that require operative vaginal delivery, the forceps and vacuum extractor are interchangeable. When the head is low in the pelvis and the occiput is anterior, vacuum extraction and forceps delivery are easy to perform and safe for the fetus. In these circumstances there is little to choose between the two instruments obstetrically, although the vacuum extractor may be more comfortable for the mother[65]. Deliveries from the midcavity of the pelvis, either with forceps or vacuum extractor, may be more complex and should never be performed by the inexperienced operator. The level and position of the fetal head may require considerable judgement to assess accurately and it is likely that some procedures fail and injuries are sustained because station and position are misjudged. As with forceps, high vacuum extractions and extractions before the cervix is fully dilated should be discouraged. Similarly, application of a vacuum cup to a high head in order to bring down the presenting part to a lower station so that delivery may be completed with forceps is not safe obstetric practice[25]. Use of the instrument in such high risk situations may be justified as an alternative to caesarean section in some circumstances[29, 30], but in general the risks to the fetus and mother make caesarean section the safer alternative.

With adequate experience, deliveries that require instrumental rotation of the head can be accomplished successfully with either forceps or vacuum extractor. However, because the cup when correctly applied does not create disproportion or interfere with the normal mechanism of internal rotation, the head is able to rotate at the most appropriate level in the pelvis. Provided the operator has been adequately trained, it would appear on balance that the vacuum extractor has advantages over forceps for rotational deliveries since it is less traumatic for the mother, requires simpler forms of analgesia and is equally safe for the baby[26]. The widely held belief that vacuum extraction is too slow to be useful when rapid delivery is required is not supported by the evidence. While the duration of the procedure from application of the instrument to the time of delivery is likely to be less with forceps, the interval between deciding on the need for instrumental assistance and the delivery itself is no greater with the vacuum extractor than with forceps[26, 38].

Maternal participation is an integral part of vacuum extraction whereas it may be less critical with forceps delivery. The birth should occur principally as a result of uterine contractions and maternal expulsive effort, complemented to a lesser extent by traction with the vacuum extractor. Measures that may reduce the strength of the contractions and maternal expulsion should be avoided. For this reason, general anaesthesia should be considered a contraindication for vacuum extraction, and epidural analgesia although not contraindicated requires a change in technique. If hypotonic uterine action develops, oxytocin administration by intravenous infusion should be instituted to enhance the contractions.

With practice, most vacuum extractions including rotational procedures can be performed with little or no analgesia whereas more powerful forms of pain relief are usually required for forceps delivery. The avoidance of general anaesthesia increases the safety of vacuum extraction. There is little doubt that the vacuum extractor is less traumatic for the mother than forceps, and that its use for operative vaginal delivery results in a substantial reduction in maternal morbidity[110]. Because the cup does not come between the presenting part and the wall of the birth canal once the head is flexed, the risk of injury to the maternal tissues should be no greater than after normal delivery. Extrapolation of the data derived from randomized controlled trials comparing vacuum extraction and forceps delivery in Britain[38, 39] has yielded interesting estimates of the extra 'costs' to women of the continued preference for forceps[81]; and because there does not appear to be any significant compensating benefits for the babies from the use of forceps, it has been suggested that the vacuum extractor should be considered the instrument of choice for operative vaginal delivery. However, other obstetric variables such as experience of the operator and selection of cases must also be taken into consideration since they are critical elements in determining whether the benefits of intervention outweigh the risks and whether vacuum extraction is preferable to forceps delivery. Enthusiasm for more widespread use of the vacuum extractor must be matched by adequate training and strict adherence to appropriate selection criteria to ensure that the procedure is safe for the infant. Since there are important differences in technique between forceps delivery and vacuum extraction, it does not follow that experience gained in one method will automatically transfer to the other. Skilled users of the obstetric forceps may benefit little from abandoning an instrument they know well in favour of the vacuum extractor unless an opportunity exists for adequate training in the new technique[34].

Despite the obvious benefits for the mother, vacuum extraction as an accepted method of operative vaginal delivery will depend largely on the effects on the newborn. Although there is not enough information available at present to judge the relative merits of the two instruments on the long term condition of the infants' sensory and intellectual functions, there is a distinct difference in short term outcomes especially in the pattern of injuries observed on the head and face[26].

The ease with which the suction cup can be applied, not always correctly, to the fetal head has been regarded as a disadvantage of the method because incorrect applications (while not harming the mother) may result in failure, seriously injure the baby and discredit the vacuum extractor[25]. On the other hand, familiarity with the equipment, knowledge of the ideal application site and correct traction technique should produce consistently good results for mother and baby.

ATTITUDES OF THE CARE-GIVERS

Because use of the obstetric forceps or vacuum extractor varies to such a great extent around the world, it is not surprising that considerable differences of opinion exist about the relative merits and disadvantages of the two instruments. Operators should appreciate that while the techniques of forceps delivery and vacuum extraction are similar, they are not identical and that experience gained with one instrument does not necessarily equate with the other. Concern has been expressed that the ease with which a vacuum cup can be applied to the fetal head allows less skilled attendants to attempt the more complex procedures[25, 146]. Even in the situation of a randomized trial, patients allocated to vacuum extraction were likely to be delivered by less experienced operators as there was a tendency for vacuum extraction to be left to the more junior obstetricians[39]. There was also a natural temptation to follow a failed vacuum extraction by an application of forceps whereas after a failed forceps, the operator tended to proceed directly to caesarean section. Attitudes and skills acquired by operators with regard to vacuum extraction will be influenced greatly by the type of exposure to the instrument and the quality of the training they receive. For this reason, all obstetricians responsible for teaching vacuum extraction and formulating training programmes should themselves have been adequately trained in the method. Structured training programmes are not common in places where forceps are the preferred instrument for assisted delivery and obstetricians in these situations must rely on self-instruction if they wish to develop expertise in the method. Fortunately it is possible to grade instrumental procedures according to the level of technical skill that is required and operators should discipline themselves to master all aspects of vacuum extraction in the straightforward deliveries before proceeding to the more complex extractions. This graduated approach will not only make the procedure safer for the infant and mother but, equally important, will help the operator to develop a sense of confidence in the method.

The extent to which a mother will accept the appearance of her baby after vacuum extraction will be influenced by the attitudes and reassurances of the staff, not only of those who perform the procedures but also of paediatricians, midwives and nurses who care for mothers and babies after birth[26]. It is important to reassure parents that a chignon will disappear in a matter of hours and that bruising and marking from the vacuum cup will leave no traces after a few days. A careless remark, however well-intentioned, may lead to unnecessary anxiety for the mother.

After completion of a randomized trial that compared forceps and vacuum extraction[39] but before the results were available, the opinions of obstetric, paediatric and midwifery staff were sought by questionnaire[65]. Medical and midwifery staff in the hospital made it clear that many of them had had very little experience of the vacuum extractor and had changed their views about the two instruments during the course of the trial. The experience of the trial and working with an advocate of the method had influenced the views of many respondents. They reported that they had a new familiarity with the vacuum extractor and a willingness to consider its use in a wider range of circumstances. Reduction in maternal trauma and pain of labour were seen as the most significant advantages of the vacuum extractor. The perceived disadvantages of the instrument were the general lack of experience in its use, the greater complexity and poor maintenance of the equipment and lack of available teaching and training. Problems of the newborn associated with the use of the vacuum extractor (such as chignon, markings and jaundice) also caused the staff some concerns.

Neonatal paediatricians and nursing staff deserve special consideration with regard to vacuum extraction; some of the babies delivered by this method and who require treatment may have sustained injuries as a result of the procedure. Not surprisingly in such circumstances, neonatal caregivers may sometimes be reluctant to accept vacuum extraction as a safe method to assist the delivery of the infant. Regular in-service instruction of the principles and technique for all medical and nursing staff involved in counselling and caring for mothers and babies should be conducted to help broaden the understanding and acceptance of vacuum extraction. Negative biases towards the instrument will be reinforced if it is used infrequently and only for complicated procedures because outcomes for the baby are more likely to be suboptimal in these circumstances. On the other hand, positive biases will be developed if the vacuum extractor is used and is seen to be used correctly for the entire range of appropriate indications.

BIBLIOGRAPHY

1. Dragotescu C C, Roman I. *Vidextractia Obstetricala*. Bucharest: Editura Academiei Republicii Populare Romine, 1962.
2. Chalmers J A. *The Ventouse: The Obstetric Vacuum Extractor*. London: Lloyd-Luke, 1971.
3. Malmstrom T. The vacuum extractor, an obstetrical instrument. *Acta Obstetricia et Gynecologica Scandinavica*. 1957; **36**, Suppl 3, 5–50.
4. Bird G C. Modification of Malmstrom's vacuum extractor. *British Medical Journal*. 1969; **3**, 526.
5. Bird G C. *Vacuum-extractor Manual*. Gothenburg: Mennox AB, 1982.
6. Halkin V. Une modification de la ventouse de Malmstrom. *Bulletin de la Societe Royale Belge Gynecologie et d'Obstetrique*. 1964; **34**, 145–50.
7. Lovset J. Modern techniques of vaginal operative delivery in cephalic presentation. *Acta Obstetricia et Gynecologica Scandinavica*. 1965; **44**, 102–6.
8. O'Neil A G B, Skull E, Michael C. A new method of traction for the vacuum cup. *Australian and New Zealand Journal of Obstetrics and Gynaecology*. 1981; **21**, 24–5.
9. Bird G C. The importance of flexion in vacuum extraction delivery. *British Journal of Obstetrics and Gynaecology*. 1976; **83**, 194–200.
10. Sjostedt J E. The vacuum extractor and forceps in obstetrics – a clinical study. *Acta Obstetricia et Gynecologica Scandinavica*. 1967; **46** (supplement 10), 1–183.
11. Party M. *Ventouses Obstétricales. La V.O.F., Ventouse Obstetricale Francaise*. Paris: Vigot Frères, 1966.
12. Saling E, Rothe J. Modifikation der Vakuumextraktionsvorrichtung. *Zeitschrift Geburtshilse und Perinatologie*. 1978; **182**, 93–5.
13. Magnin P. Ventouses obstetricales. In: *Extractions Instrumentales du Foetus*. Paris Encyclopédie Medico-Chirurgicale, 1976: Vol. 5095A50, 1–8.
14. Johanson R. Soft versus hard vacuum extractor cups. In: Chalmers I ed. *Oxford Database of Perinatal Trials*, Version 1.2, Disk Issue 5, February 1991. Record 5451.
15. Constantine G, Basu S N, Hampton N. Alternative vacuum supplies for ventouse deliveries. *British Journal of Obstetrics and Gynaecology*. 1989; **96**, 249–50.
16. Pearson M J. Alternative vacuum supplies for ventouse deliveries (letter to the editor). *British Journal of Obstetrics and Gynaecology*. 1989; **96**, 751.
17. Ott W J. Vacuum extraction. *Obstetrical and Gynecological Survey*. 1975; **30**, 643–9.
18. Wider J A, Erez S, Steer C M. An evaluation of the vacuum extractor in a series of 201 cases. *American Journal of Obstetrics and Gynecology*. 1967; **98**, 24–31.
19. Lasbrey A H, Orchard C D, Crichton D. A study of the relative merits and scope for vacuum extraction as opposed to forceps delivery. *South African Journal of Obstetrics and Gynaecology*. 1964; **2**, 1–3.
20. Rydberg E. *The Mechanism of Labour*. Springfield: Charles C Thomas, 1954: 1–180.
21. Caldwell W E, Moloy H C, d'Esopo D A. A roentgenologic study of the mechanism of engagement of the fetal head. *American Journal of Obstetrics and Gynecology*. 1934; **28**, 824–41.
22. Lewis T L T, Chamberlain G V P. Anatomy of the normal female pelvis and the fetal skull. In: Lewis T L T, Chamberlain G V F eds. *Obstetrics by Ten Teachers*. London: Edward Arnold, 1990: 18–24.
23. Lindgren L. The causes of foetal head moulding in labour. *Acta Obstetricia et Gynecologica Scandinavica*. 1960; **39**, 46–62.
24. Malmstrom T, Jansson I. Use of the vacuum extractor. *Clinical Obstetrics and Gynecology*. 1965; **8**, 893–913.
25. Bird G C. The use of the vacuum extractor. *Clinics in Obstetrics and Gynaecology*. 1982; **9**, 641–61.
26. Vacca A, Keirse M J N C. Instrumental vaginal delivery. In Chalmers I, Enkin M, Keirse M J N C eds. *Effective Care in Pregnancy and Childbirth*.

Oxford: Oxford University Press, 1989: 1216–33.

27. Bergsjo P, Schmidt E, Pusch D. Differences in the reported frequencies of some obstetrical interventions in Europe. *British Journal of Obstetrics and Gynaecology*. 1983; 90, 628–32.

28. Lomas J, Enkin M. Variations in operative delivery-rates. In: Chalmers I, Enkin M, Keirse M J N C eds. *Effective Care in Pregnancy and Childbirth*. Oxford: Oxford University Press, 1989: 1182–95.

29. Chukwudebelu W O. Vacuum extraction before full cervical dilatation. *International Surgery*. 1978; 63, 89–90.

30. Chalmers I, Richard M. Intervention and causal inference in obstetric practice. In: Chard T, Richard M eds. *Benefits and Hazards of the New Obstetrics*. London: Heinemann, 1977: 34–61.

31. O'Driscoll K, Jackson R J A, Gallagher J T. Active management of labour and cephalopelvic disproportion. *Journal of Obstetrics and Gynaecology of the British Commonwealth*. 1970; 77, 385–9.

32. de Villiers J N, Bornman J J. Vacuum extraction – a review and assessment. *South African Medical Journal*. 1963; 37, 574–82.

33. Bird G C. The use of the Malmstrom vacuum extractor in operative obstetrics. *Australian and New Zealand Journal of Obstetrics and Gynaecology*. 1966; 6, 242–7.

34. Iffy L, Lancet M, Kessler I. The vacuum extractor. In: Iffy L, Charles D eds. *Operative Perinatology*. New York: Macmillan, 1984: 582–94.

35. Huntingford P J. The vacuum extractor in the treatment of delay in first stage of labour. *The Lancet*. 1961; 1, 1054–7.

36. Simons E G, Philpott R H. The vacuum extractor. *Tropical Doctor*. 1973; 3, 34–7.

37. Roberts I F, Stone M. Fetal haemorrhage: complications of the vacuum extractor after fetal blood sampling. *American Journal of Obstetrics and Gynecology*. 1978; 132, 109.

38. Johanson R, Pusey J, Livera J, Jones P. North Staffordshire/Wigan assisted delivery trial. *British Journal of Obstetrics and Gynaecology*. 1989; 96, 537–44.

39. Vacca A, Grant A, Wyatt G, Chalmers I. Portsmouth operative delivery trial: a comparison of vacuum extraction and forceps delivery. *British Journal of Obstetrics and Gynaecology*. 1983; 90, 1107–12.

40. Thiery M. Fetal hemorrhage following blood samplings and use of vacuum extractor (letter to editor). *American Journal of Obstetrics and Gynecology*. 1979; 134, 231.

41. Chamberlain G. Forceps and vacuum extraction. *Clinics in Obstetrics and Gynaecology*. 1980; 7, 511–27.

42. Greis J B, Bieniarz J, Scommegna A. Comparison of maternal and fetal effects of vacuum extraction with forceps or caesarean section. *Obstetrics and Gynecology*. 1981; 57, 571–7.

43. Sleep J, Roberts J, Chalmers I. Care during the second stage of labour. In: Chalmers I, Enkin M, Keirse M J N C eds. *Effective Care in Pregnancy and Childbirth*. Oxford: Oxford University Press, 1989: 1129–44.

44. Morgan B M, Bulpitt C J, Clifton P, Lewish P J. Analgesia and satisfaction in childbirth (The Queen Charlotte's One Thousand Mother Survey). *The Lancet*. 1982; 2, 808–10.

45. Willcourt R J. Uterine activity in labour. In: Studd J ed. *Progress in Obstetrics and Gynaecology Vol 3*. Edinburgh: Churchill Livingstone, 1983: 113–27.

46. Stewart K S. The second stage. In: Studd J ed. *Progress in Obstetrics and Gynaecology Vol 4*. Edinburgh: Churchill Livingstone, 1984: 197–216.

47. Crowther C, Enkin M, Keirse M J N C, Brown I. Monitoring the progress of labour. In: Chalmers I, Enkin M, Keirse M J N C eds. *Effective Care in Pregnancy and Childbirth*. Oxford: Oxford University Press, 1989: 833–45.

48. Saunders N J St.G, Spiby H, Gilbert L, Fraser R B *et al*. Oxytocin infusion during second stage of labour in primiparous women using epidural analgesia: a randomised double blind placebo controlled trial. *British Medical Journal*. 1989; 299, 1423–6.

49. Hendricks C H, Brenner W E, Kraus G. Normal cervical dilatation pattern in late pregnancy and labour. *American Journal of Obstetrics and Gynecology*. 1970; 106, 1065–82.

50. Duignan N M, Studd J W W, Hughes A O. Characteristics of normal labour in different racial groups. *British Journal of Obstetrics and Gynaecology*. 1975; 82, 593–601.

51. Philpott R H, Castle W M. Cervicographs in the management of labour in primigravidae: 1, the alert line for detecting abnormal labour. *Journal of Obstetrics and Gynaecology of the British Commonwealth*. 1972; 79, 592–8.

52. Bird G C. Cervicographic management of labour in primigravidae and multigravidae with vertex presentation. *Tropical Doctor*. 1978; 8, 78–84.

53. Studd, J W W. Partograms and nomograms in the management of primigravid labour. *British Medical Journal*. 1973; 4, 451–5.

54. Derham R J, Crowhurst J, Crowther C. The second stage of labour: durational dilemmas. *Australian and New Zealand Journal of Obstetrics and Gynaecology*. 1991; 31, 31–6.

55. Chalmers I, Garcia J, Post S. Hospital policies for labour and delivery. In: Chalmers I, Enkin M,

Keirse M J N C eds. *Effective Care in Pregnancy and Childbirth.* Oxford: Oxford University Press, 1989: 815–19.

56. O'Driscoll K, Meagher D. *Active Management of Labour.* London: W B Saunders, 1980.

57. O'Driscoll K, Jackson R J A, Gallagher J T. Prevention of prolonged labour. *British Medical Journal.* 1969; **2**, 477–80.

58. Crichton D. A reliable method of establishing the level of the fetal head in obstetrics. *South African Medical Journal.* 1974; **48**, 784–7.

59. Philpott R H. The recognition of cephalopelvic disproportion. *Clinics in Obstetrics and Gynaecology.* 1982; **9**, 609–24.

60. Myerscough P R. Intranatal welfare of the infant. In: Myerscough P R ed. *Munro Kerr's Operative Obstetrics.* London: Baillière Tindall, 1982: 21–35.

61. Stewart K S. 1977 M.D. Thesis, University of Edinburgh. Cited in: Myerscough P R ed. *Munro Kerr's Operative Obstetrics.* London: Baillière Tindall, 1982: 32.

62. Bird G C, Bal J S. Subcutaneous symphysiotomy in association with the vacuum extractor. *Journal of Obstetrics and Gynaecology of the British Commonwealth.* 1967; **74**, 266–9.

63. Gebbie D. Symphysiotomy. *Clinics in Obstetrics and Gynaecology.* 1982; **9**, 663–83.

64. Lancet M, Borenstein R. Vaginal instrumental extraction – changing trends. In: Iffy L, Charles D eds. *Operative Perinatology.* New York: Macmillan, 1984: 554–61.

65. Garcia J, Anderson J, Vacca A, Elbourne D, Grant A. Chalmers I. Views of women and their medical and midwifery attendants about instrumental delivery using vacuum extraction and forceps. *Journal of Psychosomatic Obstetrics and Gynaecology.* 1985; **4**, 1–9.

66. Moolgaoker A. A safe alternative to caesarean section? *Journal of Obstetrics and Gynaecology of the British Commonwealth.* 1970; **77**, 1077–87.

67. Aguero O, Alvarez H. Fetal injuries due to the vacuum extractor. *Obstetrics and Gynecology.* 1962; **19**, 212–17.

68. Lange P. Clinical experience with the vacuum extractor. *Danish Medical Bulletin.* 1961; **8**, 11–16.

69. Thiery M, Van Den Broecke R, Kermans G, Parewijck W *et al.* A randomised study of two cups for vacuum extraction. *Journal of Perinatal Medicine.* 1987; **15**, 129–36.

70. Johanson R. O'Neil versus Malmstrom vacuum extraction. In: Chalmers I ed. *Oxford Database of Perinatal Trials,* Version 1.2, Disk Issue 5, February 1991. Record 3795.

71. Carmody F, Grant A, Somchiwong M. Vacuum extraction: a randomised comparison of the New Generation cup with the original Bird cup. *Journal of Perinatal Medicine.* 1986; **14**, 95–100.

72. Dell D L, Sightler S E, Plauche W C. Soft cup vacuum extraction: a comparison of outlet delivery. *Obstetrics and Gynecology.* 1985; **66**, 624–8.

73. Johanson R. Silastic versus Mityvac vacuum extraction. In: Chalmers I ed. *Oxford Database of Perinatal Trials,* Version 1.2, Disk Issue 5, February 1991. Record 3258.

74. Berkhus M D, Ramamurthy R S, O'Connor P S, Brown K, Hayashi R H. Cohort study of Silastic obstetric vacuum cup deliveries: 1, safety of the instrument. *Obstetrics and Gynecology.* 1985; **66**, 503–9.

75. Hastie S J, Maclean A B. Comparison of the use of the Silastic obstetric vacuum extractor to Kielland's forceps. *Asia-Oceania Journal of Obstetrics and Gynaecology.* 1986; **12**, 63–8.

76. Svigos J M, Cave D G, Vigneswaran R, Resch A, Christiansen J. Silastic cup vacuum extractor or forceps: A comparative study. *Asia-Oceania Journal of Obstetrics and Gynaecology.* 1990; **16**, 323–7.

77. Hammarstrom M, Csemiczky G, Belfrage P. Comparison between the conventional Malmstrom extractor and a new extractor with Silastic cup. *Acta Obstetricia et Gynecologica Scandinavica.* 1986; **65**, 791–2.

78. Cohn M, Barclay C, Fraser R, Zaklama M, Johanson R, Anderson D, Walker C. A multicentre randomised trial comparing delivery with a silicone rubber cup and rigid metal vacuum extractor cups. *British Journal of Obstetrics and Gynaecology.* 1989; **96**, 545–51.

79. Hofmeyr G J, Gobetz L, Sonnendecker E W W, Turner M J. New design rigid and soft vacuum extractor cups: a preliminary comparison of traction forces. *British Journal of Obstetrics and Gynaecology.* 1990; **97**, 681–5.

80. Halme J. The vacuum extractor for obstetric delivery. *Clinical Obstetrics and Gynecology.* 1982; **25**, 167–75.

81. Chalmers J A, Chalmers I. The obstetric vacuum extractor is the instrument of first choice for operative vaginal delivery. *British Journal of Obstetrics and Gynaecology.* 1989; **96**, 505–6.

82. Stewart P. Posture in labour. In: Studd J ed. *Progress in Obstetrics and Gynaecology Vol 8.* Edinburgh: Churchill Livingstone, 1990: 86–96.

83. Humphrey M D, Chang A, Wood E C, Morgan S, Hownslow D. A decrease of fetal pH during the second stage of labour, when conducted in dorsal position. *Journal of Obstetrics and Gynaecology of the British Commonwealth.* 1974; **81**, 600–602.

84. Larsen J V. The vacuum extractor and the left

lateral position. *South African Medical Journal.* 1977; **51**, 492.

85.   O'Neil G. How to get the best results from vacuum extraction. *Proceedings from the Sixth Congress of the Federation of the Asia-Oceania Perinatal Societies.* 1990: 156.

86.   Pearse W H. Forceps versus spontaneous delivery. *Clinical Obstetrics and Gynecology.* 1965; **8**, 813–21.

87.   Chalmers J A. The management of malrotation of the occiput. *Journal of Obstetrics and Gynaecology of the British Commonwealth.* 1968; **75**, 889–91.

88.   Broekhuizen F F, Washington J M, Johnson F, Hamilton P R. Vacuum extraction versus forceps delivery: indications and complications, 1979 to 1984. *Obstetrics and Gynecology.* 1987; **69**, 338–42.

89.   Chukwudebelu W O. The vacuum extractor in difficult labor. *International Surgery.* 1977; **62**, 89–90.

90.   Ehlers N, Jensen I K, Hansen K B. Retinal haemorrhages in the newborn – a comparison of delivery by forceps and by vacuum extractor. *Acta Ophthalmologica.* 1974; **52**, 73–82.

91.   Nyirjesy I, Hawks B L, Falls H C, Munsat T L, Pierce W E. A comparative clinical study of the vacuum extractor and forceps. *American Journal of Obstetrics and Gynecology.* 1963; **85**, 1071–82.

92.   Punnonen R, Aro P, Kuukankorpi A. Pystynen P. Fetal and maternal effects of forceps and vacuum extraction. *British Journal of Obstetrics and Gynaecology.* 1986; **93**, 1132–5.

93.   Schenker J G, Serr D M. Comparative study of delivery by vacuum extractor and forceps. *American Journal of Obstetrics and Gynecology.* 1967; **98**, 32–9.

94.   Maryniak G M, Frank J B. Clinical assessment of the Kobayashi vacuum extractor. *Obstetrics and Gynecology.* 1984; **64**, 431–5.

95.   Plauche W C. Fetal cranial injuries related to delivery with the Malmstrom vacuum extractor. *Obstetrics and Gynecology.* 1979; **53**, 750–7.

96.   Hoult I J, MacLennan A H, Carrie L E S. Lumbar epidural analgesia in labour: relation to fetal malposition and instrumental delivery. *British Medical Journal.* 1977; **1**, 14–16.

97.   Jouppila R, Jouppila P, Karinen J M, Hollmen A. Segmental epidural analgesia in labour: related to the progress of labour, fetal malposition and instrumental delivery. *Acta Obstetricia et Gynecologica Scandinavica.* 1979; **58**, 135–9.

98.   Kaminski H M, Stafl A. Aiman J. The effect of epidural analgesia on the frequency of instrumental obstetric delivery. *Obstetrics and Gynecology.* 1987; **69**, 770–3.

99.   Lancet M. Use of the vacuum extractor. *British Medical Journal.* 1963; **1**, 165–9.

100. Blunt A. The place of the vacuum extractor in obstetric practice. *Australian and New Zealand Journal of Obstetrics and Gynaecology.* 1964; **4**, 156–9.

101. Svenningsen L. Birth progression and traction forces developed under vacuum extraction after slow or rapid application of suction. *European Journal of Obstetrical and Gynecological Reproductive Biology.* 1987; **26**, 105–12.

102. Moolgaoker A S, Ahmed S O S, Payne P R. A comparison of different methods of instrumental delivery based on electronic measurements of compression and traction. *Obstetrics and Gynecology.* 1979; **54**, 299–309.

103. Saling E, Hartung M. Analyses of tractive forces during the application of vacuum extraction. *Journal of Perinatal Medicine.* 1973; **1**, 245–51.

104. Duchon M A, De Mund M A, Brown R H. Laboratory comparison of modern vacuum extractors. *Obstetrics and Gynecology.* 1988; **71**, 155–8.

105. Issel E P. Zur mechanischen einwirkung der geburtshilflichen Zange auf den fetalen Schadel. *Zentralblatt fur Gynakologie.* 1977; **99**, 487–97.

106. Awon M P. The vacuum extractor – experimental demonstration of distortion of the foetal skull. *Journal of Obstetrics and Gynaecology of the British Commonwealth.* 1964; **71**, 634–6.

107. Pearse W H. Electronic recording of forceps delivery. *American Journal of Obstetrics and Gynecology.* 1963; **86**, 43–9.

108. Fahmy K. Uterine rupture and vacuum extraction. *International Journal of Gynecology and Obstetrics.* 1976; **14**, 509–12.

109. Rachagan S P, Raman S, Galasundram G, Balakrishnam S. Rupture of the pregnant uterus – a 21 year review. *Australian and New Zealand Journal of Obstetrics and Gynaecology.* 1991; **31**, 37–40.

110. Johanson R. Vacuum extraction vs forceps delivery. In: Chalmers I ed. *Oxford Database of Perinatal Trials*, Version 1.2, Disk Issue 5, February 1991. Record 3256.

111. Carmody F, Grant A M, Mutch L, Vacca A, Chalmers I. Follow-up of babies delivered in a randomised controlled comparison of vacuum extraction and forceps delivery. *Acta Obstetricia et Gynecologica Scandinavica.* 1986; **65**, 763–6.

112. Bjerre I, Dahlin K. The long-term development of children delivered by vacuum extraction. *Developmental Medicine and Child Neurology.* 1974; **16**, 378–81.

113. Livnat E J, Fejgin M, Scommegna A, Bieniarz J, Burd L. Neonatal acid-base balance in spontaneous and instrumental vaginal deliveries. *American Journal of Obstetrics and Gynecology.* 1978; **52**, 549–51.

114. Derom R, Thiery M, Lybeer E. The lactate-pyruvate balance in relation to vacuum extraction. *Journal of Obstetrics and Gynaecology of the British Commonwealth*. 1965; **72**, 892–5.

115. Thiery M, van Kets H, Derom R. Recording of tractive power in vacuum extractions (letter to editor). *Journal of Perinatal Medicine* 1973; **1**, 291.

116. Leijon I. Neurology and behaviour of newborn infants delivered by vacuum extraction on maternal indication. *Acta Paediatrica Scandinavica*. 1980; **69**, 625–31.

117. Katz Z, Lancet M, Dgani R, Ben-Hur H, Zalel Y. The beneficial effect of vacuum extraction on the fetus. *Acta Obstetricia et Gynecologica Scandinavica*. 1982; **61**, 337–40.

118. O'Grady J P. *Modern Instrumental Delivery*. Baltimore: Williams and Wilkins, 1988.

119. Levin S, Janive J, Mintz K, Kreisler C, Romem M, Klutznik A, Feingold M and Insler V. Diagnostic and prognostic value of retinal haemorrhages in the neonate. *Obstetrics and Gynecology*. 1980; **55**, 309–14.

120. von Barsewisch B. *Perinatal retinal haemorrhages*. Berlin, Heidelberg, New York: Springer-Verlag, 1979.

121. Schenker J G, Gombos G M. Retinal haemorrhage in the newborn. *Obstetrics and Gynecology*. 1966; **27**, 521–4.

122. Egge K, Lyng G, Maltau J M. Effect of instrumental delivery on the frequency and severity of retinal haemorrhages in the newborn. *Acta Obstetricia et Gynecologica Scandinavica*. 1981; **60**, 153–5.

123. Fall O, Ryden G, Finnstrom K, Finnstrom O, Leijon I. Forceps or vacuum extraction? A comparison of effects on the newborn infant. *Acta Obstetricia et Gynecologica Scandinavica*. 1986; **65**, 75–80.

124. Svenningsen L, Lindemann R, Eidal K, Jensen O. Neonatal retinal haemorrhages and neurobehaviour related to tractive force in vacuum extraction. *Acta Obstetricia et Gynecologica Scandinavica*. 1987; **66**, 165–9.

125. Boon W H. Vacuum extraction in obstetrics (letter to editor). *Lancet*. 1961; **2**, 662.

126. Baerthlein W C, Moodley S, Stinson S K. Comparison of maternal and neonatal morbidity in midforceps delivery and midpelvis vacuum extraction. *Obstetrics and Gynecology*. 1986; **67**, 594–7.

127. Thiery M. Obstetric vacuum extraction. In: Wynn R M ed. *Obstetrics and Gynecology Annual* Norwalk: Appleton-Century-Crofts, 1985: 73–111.

128. Plauche W C. Subgaleal hematoma, a complication of instrumental delivery. *Journal of the*

American Medical Association. 1980; **244**, 1597–8.

129. Robinson R J, Rossiter M A. Massive subaponeurotic haemorrhage in babies of African origin. *Archives of the Diseases of Childhood*. 1968; **43**, 684–7.

130. Ahuja G L, Willoughby M L N, Kerr M M, Hutchison J H. Massive subaponeurotic haemorrhage in infants born by vacuum extraction. *British Medical Journal*. 1969; **3**, 743–5.

131. Williams M F, Jacobs M, Moosa A. Subaponeurotic haemmorhage of the newborn. *South African Medical Journal*. 1977; **52**, 176–8.

132. Campbell N, Harvey D, Norman A P. Increased frequency of neonatal jaundice in a maternity hospital. *British Medical Journal*. 1975; **2**, 548–52.

133. Friedman E A, Sachtleben M R. Neonatal jaundice in association with oxytocin stimulation of labour and operative delivery. *British Medical Journal*. 1976; **1**, 198–9.

134. Fenichel G M, Webster D L, Wong W K T. Intracranial hemorrhage in the term newborn. *Archives of Neurology*. 1984; **41**, 30–4.

135. Jeannin P, Afschrift M, Voet D, Vanderkerckhove F. Thiery M, Defoort P. Derom R. Cranial ultrasound after forceful midpelvis vacuum extraction at term. *Journal of Perinatal Medicine*. 1984; **12**, 319–23.

136. Tudehope D I, Vacca A. Traumatic injuries to the nervous system. In: Levene M I, Bennett M J, Punt J eds. *Fetal and Neonatal Neurology and Neurosurgery*. London: Churchill Livingstone, 1988: 393–404.

137. Ludwig B, Brand M, Brockerhoff P. Postpartum CT examination of the heads of full term infants. *Neuroradiology*. 1980; **20**, 145–54.

138. Lahat E, Schiffer J, Heyman E, Dolphin Z, Starinski R. Acute subdural hemorrhage: uncommon complication of vacuum extraction delivery. *European Journal of Obstetrical and Gynaecological Reproductive Biology*. 1987; **25**, 255–8.

139. Benedetti T J, Gabbe S G. Shoulder dystocia, a complication of fetal macrosomia and prolonged second stage of labour with mid-pelvic delivery. *Obstetrics and Gynecology*. 1978; **52**, 526–9.

140. Hunter D J S and Keirse M J N C. Gestational diabetes. In: Chalmers I, Enkin M, Keirse M J N C eds. *Effective Care in Pregnancy and Childbirth*. Oxford: Oxford University Press, 1989: 403–10.

141. Acker D B, Sachs B P, Friedman E A. Risk factors for shoulder dystocia. *Obstetrics and Gynecology*. 1985; **66**, 762–8.

142. Hunter D J S. Diabetes in pregnancy. In: Chalmers I, Enkin M, Keirse M J N C eds. *Effective Care in Pregnancy and Childbirth*. Oxford: Oxford University Press, 1989: 578–93.

143. Acker D B, Sachs B P, Friedman E A. Risk factors

for shoulder dystocia in the average weight infant. *Obstetrics and Gynecology.* 1986; **67**, 614–18.

144. Hofmeyr G J. Suspected fetopelvic disproportion. In: Chalmers I, Enkin M, Keirse M J N C eds. *Effective Care in Pregnancy and Childbirth.* Oxford: Oxford University Press, 1989: 493–8.

145. Gross T L, Sokol R J, Williams P and Thompson K. Shoulder dystocia: a fetal-physician risk. *American Journal of Obstetrics and Gynecology.* 1987; **156**, 1408–14.

146. McFarland L V, Raskin M, Daling J R and Benedetti T J. Erb/Duchenne's palsy: a consequence of fetal macrosomia and method of delivery. *Obstetrics and Gynecology.* 1986; **68**, 784–8.

147. Elliott J P, Garite T J, Freeman R K, McQuown D S, Patel J M. Ultrasonic prediction of fetal macrosomia in diabetic patients. *Obstetrics and Gynecology.* 1982; **60**, 159–62.

148. Gabbe S G, Mestman J H, Freeman R K, Anderson G V, Lowensohn R I. Management and outcome of class A diabetes mellitus, *American Journal of Obstetrics and Gynecology.* 1977; **127**, 465–9.

149. Chang Y L. Shoulder dystocia. *Clinical Obstetrics and Gynecology.* 1987; 30, 77–82.

150. Sandberg E C. The Zavanelli Maneuver: a potentially revolutionary method for the resolution of shoulder dystocia. *American Journal of Obstetrics and Gynecology.* 1985; **152**, 479–82.

151. Benedetti T J. Managing shoulder dystocia. *Contemporary Ob/Gyn.* 1979; **14**, 33–8.

152. Holman M S. A new manoeuvre for delivery of an impacted shoulder, based on a mechanical analysis. *South African Medical Journal (Supplement – South African Journal of Obstetrics and Gynaecology).* 1963; **37**, 247–9.

153. Varner M W. Neuropsychiatric sequelae of midforceps deliveries. *Clinics in Perinatology.* 1983; **10**, 455–60.

154. Stanley F. Perinatal risk factors in the cerebral palsies. In: Stanley F. Alberman E eds. *The Epidemiology of the Cerebral Palsies.* Oxford: Blackwell Scientific Publications. 1984: 98–115.

155. Bryce R, Stanley F, Blair E. The effects of intrapartum care on the risks of impairments in childhood. In: Chalmers I, Enkin M, Keirse M J N C eds. *Effective Care in Pregnancy and Childbirth.* Oxford: Oxford University Press, 1989: 1313–21.

156. Blennow G, Svenningsen N W, Gustafson B, Sunden B, Cronquist S. Neonatal and prospective follow-up study of infants delivered by vacuum extraction (VE). *Acta Obstetricia et Gynecologica Scandinavica.* 1977; **56**, 189–94.

157. Bowes W A, Bowes C. Current role of the midforceps operation. *Clinical Obstetrics and Gynecology.* 1980; **23**, 549–57.

158. Editorial. Kielland's forceps or Ventouse – a comparison. *Obstetrical and Gynecological Survey.* 1989; **44**, 373–4.

159. Editorial. A safe alternative to caesarean section? *Obstetrical and Gynecological Survey.* 1971; **26**, 515–18.

160. Healy D L, Laufe L E. Survey of obstetric forceps training in North America in 1981. *American Journal of Obstetrics and Gynecology.* 1985; **151**, 54–8.

161. Opit L J. Selwood T S. Caesarean-section rates in Australia. *Medical Journal of Australia.* 1979; **2**, 706–9.

162. Editorial. Kielland's forceps. *British Medical Journal.* 1979; **1**, 362–3.

163. Chalmers I. Evaluating the effects of care during pregnancy and childbirth. In: Chalmers I, Enkin M, Keirse M J N C eds. *Effective Care in Pregnancy and Childbirth.* Oxford: Oxford University Press, 1989: 3–38.

INDEX